PROVINGS

by

RAJAN SANKARAN

HOMOEOPATHIC MEDICAL PUBLISHERS
20, Station Road, Santa Cruz (W), Mumbai-400054.

First Edition : 1998

ISBN-81-900810-8-X

Realised by
Brihat Consultants, Pondicherry - 605 001

Printed at
Surya Graphics, Kottivakkam, Chennai - 600 041

Published by
HOMOEOPATHIC MEDICAL PUBLISHERS
20, Station Road, Santa Cruz (W), Mumbai-400054.

ACKNOWLEDGEMENT

This book is here because of the working together of various dedicated people. My contribution is only to have brought them together and to have coordinated the provings.

The reader of the book must thank the provers, who will remain anonymous and who gave so much to Homoeopathy.

The provings were transcribed and put in the present format by Dr. Rashmi Jaising. Her painstaking and accurate work is primarily responsible for the standard of this book.

Mr. T.D. Antony has been very patient and dedicated in the typing of this book.

Last but not least, the spark provided by Dr. Jurgen Becker and Jeremy Sherr is largely responsible for this work and to them the profession remains indebted.

To all these people, on behalf of the readers and myself, I say thank you.

NOTE

After each symptom information is provided in brackets as follows, for example [A/m/2,3/i]:

- "A" denotes the prover.
- "m" or "f" denotes the sex of the prover.
- 2,3 implies that the prover experienced the symptom on the third day of the second week of the proving.
- "i" denotes that the prover experienced the symptom after one dose of the remedy.

In all the provings capital letters have been used to denote the provers, except for the seminar provings of *Lac humanum* and *Coca-Cola* where numbers are used instead.

Where the prime sign has been used, for example "B' ", it implies that the prover did not take the dose.

"S" implies that the prover smelt the dose and did not take it orally.

Where information about any of the above was not available the " * " has been used. This is true especially in the seminar provings which were not supervised.

Where the rubrics are put:

- in ordinary type : they carry one mark;
- in *italics* : they carry two marks and,
- in **bold** type : they carry three marks.

CONTENTS

INTRODUCTION

Provings have been and still are the bedrock of the science and practice of Homoeopathy, ever since the first proving of *Cinchona* by Hahnemann in 1796. After his proving of nearly a hundred remedies, there was a lull for many decades. Of course, valuable new remedies were incorporated into the Materia Medica through some provings that were carried out in this time, *Lachesis*, *Naja* and *Tuberculinum*, to name just a few. Also, smaller, less detailed provings of other remedies were done, but these were of limited value: they did not seem to bring out the full features of the remedies. In short, it seems that provings were not given the importance that they enjoyed in the Hahnemannian era, and so the number of significant and reliable additions to our Materia Medica were few.

However, in the last decade, and more so, in the last five years, the scenario has changed remarkably; there has been a radical increase in the number of provings, worldwide. Among the first to initiate the new set of provings was Dr. Jurgen Becker from Frieburg, Germany. He certainly brought Homoeopathy out of the closet, and changed our perception of each remedial substance from being a mere dry collection of data into a living, colourful, throbbing spirit. He devised a new and revolutionary method of provings, that involved making an entire group of persons take a dose of the remedy, a few days before or even during a seminar, and then discussing the effects of the dose during the seminar. He began these provings at his seminars at Bad Boll. They were usually very productive in terms of symptomatology, especially in the emotional sphere in the dreams, which gave an idea of the inner processes of the substance. While these dream provings were received with a lot of enthusiasm by some, others, especially the more official ones, dismissed them as mere figments of the imagination, and it is possible that there is some truth in the latter presumption.

Later, Jeremy Sherr started his proving of *Scorpion* in England, in a detailed and Hahnemannian fashion; however, in subsequent provings, he went on to adopt a method midway between the traditional Hahnemannian and the neo-provings of Jurgen Becker.

My own personal contact with Jurgen Becker inspired me to start group-provings in Bombay, especially after I had noted seemingly indifferent results with the Hahnemannian method. At a joint seminar in Bombay in 1988, Jurgen Becker and I conducted a dream proving of *Naja*. I was impressed by the effect that the dose had on the collective group consciousness, and how, when taken collectively, the effect of the dose seemed to multiply and become much more prominent than when given on an individual basis. I, too, began to work with this method, and conducted several group-provings, such as *Ferrum*, *Calcarea silicata*, *Iodum*, and *Ringworm*. While these provings did reveal the characteristic features of the remedies, especially their mental, emotional states, there seemed to be something lacking in terms of solid data. This solid data was needed to systematize these group-provings, and here the Hahnemannian protocol of carefully detailing mental emotional and characteristic, peculiar physical symptoms, came in. My proving method, too, approximated the halfway method, as followed by Jeremy Sherr.

While I continued to conduct the provings in groups to enhance the effects of the dose, I also began to pay attention, at the same time, to the symptoms of the provers that were peculiar and characteristic. Now, we could ensure reliable, solid data on which to base prescriptions rather than generate a mere concept of the remedy, which had been the danger of provings as I had done them earlier. Such concepts could be flexible and theoretical in terms of understanding the remedy, and could be stretched to fit in cases. Of course, in these provings too, the great deal of mental symptoms and dreams predominated, and the same is reflected in this book. The proving groups consisted of volunteers, usually either practising homoeopaths or students of Homoeopathy in any number between five and twenty-five. The provers first met with me as a group, and during this meeting we discussed the purpose of the proving. Also, each prover talked about his intention in doing the provings, in this way revealing something about his personality. A dose of the remedy in the 30 C potency was distributed to all provers. In all provings, I initially gave only a single dose of the remedy to all provers, excepting for the proving of *Lac caprinum* where the provers took four doses serially. Usually, after the first dose, I did not repeat the dose for the next four days at least, and repeated it only if the prover did not apparently experience any symptoms, or the symptoms had ceased. I consider even a single dream or an out of the ordinary experience to be a symptom. The provers were asked to observe their symptoms, and it has been my observation that even those who do not take the proving dose will experience some symptoms. Such symptoms have been reported in this book. Mention has been made about these provers at the beginning of each proving. Each prover was asked to observe and note:

- All physical symptoms with exact modalities.
- All emotional symptoms with exact feelings.
- All dreams with exact feelings.
- All phenomena and incidents that happened around him during the period of the proving.
- Observations of others around him about changes in his state during the proving.
- The persons the prover met or was impressed by, the kind of movies or books that attracted him, his dress style, manner of talking, working, etc. These may initially seem to the prover to be a part of his own nature but when, later, different provers compare their experiences, they note astonishing similarities.

After the first group meeting, the provers met with me individually at the end of the first week. I made note of their symptoms, and also recorded all that they had said on video. This is preferable since their exact expressions can be recorded. If any of the provers had any problems, in terms of a troublesome symptom, they were asked to get in touch with me so that the same could be treated. At the end of the second week, the provers met as a group again, and discussed the effects of the remedy. This was repeated at the end of three or four weeks, or whenever I felt that the proving had reached a deep enough level to reveal the deepest feelings of the remedy, during which time the proving was discussed in its entirety. At this stage, I have often noted, that the experience of one prover may stimulate the memory of another and this can create a very strong effect in the room. In this way then the whole feeling and state is brought up and more clearly defined. Then this is discussed further with various other phenomena, and the whole problem and conflict within the remedy is exposed. It is only at this time that I revealed the name of the remedy to the provers, and we had a further discussion with reference to what was already known about the remedy or its source, so that a deeper understanding was reached. The provers, were asked to continue to observe and note symptoms and to report the same to me.

The provings reported in this book were all conducted in Bombay, except for the proving of *Coca-Cola* which was conducted at my seminar in San Francisco in 1994. The latter, and the proving of *Lac humanum*, conducted at my Bombay seminar in 1995, are the only seminar provings I have included here. Also, in all the provings, only I knew the name of the remedy being proved, except for the proving of *Ocimum sanctum* where even I did not know what was being proved. The symptoms that are reported here are an almost exact transcription of the video recordings that were done when the provers met with me individually.

Such a method of proving has distinct advantages. First, as I have already mentioned, the effects of the substance seem to multiply when it is given to a group, rather than to a set of individuals having no contact with each other. Various experiments that I have conducted have convinced me of the phenomenon of "group consciousness". Secondly, when the group meets to discuss the proving at its conclusion, many things hitherto unnoticed and dismissed by individual provers as being irrelevant or mere coincidences, are seen to actually be important parts of the proving. Thirdly, by giving importance to dreams and emotional phenomena, together with incidences and happenings synchronous with the provings and provers, one can draw some very valuable inferences, especially if these are considered in taking into account the rest of the proving.

I have attempted, as far as has been possible, to conduct and report the provings with the minimum error and subjectivity. This I have done in the following ways. Firstly, the name of the substance being proved was kept from all the provers. This minimizes the danger of certain provers creating symptoms out of their own imaginations, and going off on their own tangent. I must admit, however, that I have not seen this phenomenon very often. Secondly, the provers were given strict instructions not to discuss, amongst themselves, their symptoms or experiences outside of the group meetings. Thirdly, when the provers were reporting their symptoms, I have recorded the symptoms both mental and physical that were spontaneously reported by them and also tried to elicit the characteristic symptoms, especially the feelings in the mental and emotional spheres, as well as the dreams. This I have done by simply probing into what was being reported, without myself prompting or suggesting anything to the provers, as is done in the process of case-taking.

In presenting the proving, I have deliberately left out any summary or conclusions. Although at the end of each proving, we did discuss and connect proving data to the substance itself, I believe these to be my own ideas, and do not wish that readers get fixated to my views of the proving. The reason is that while sometimes, such links are clear and revealing, it is always possible that one may try to force such a link and take poetic license with the proving data. The danger of the whole proving matter being presented by a person wearing coloured glasses is similar to the danger of case-taking done with prejudice. The need to be objective and faithful is paramount. I have therefore tried, as far as possible, to be puritan with the proving data; in fact most symptoms are recorded here verbatim as the provers have reported them. In creating the rubrics, as well, I have stuck to what the provers said, rather than to my understanding of the remedy or any "themes" that seemed to emerge during the proving.

The provings have been arranged under theme headings for the convenience of the reader. Here I strongly warn the reader to avoid concentrating on these and simply glossing over the rest of the proving. The theme headings are not revealing of the symptomatology of the remedy; they are merely broad and general headings under which symptoms have been grouped so that reading becomes less cumbersome. In fact, many very important mental symptoms and dreams may be found under the heading, "Miscellaneous"; this was deliberately done to avoid creating more specific themes. Our Materia Medicas are full of peculiar and characteristic symptoms, and in emphasizing abstractions and themes, there lies the danger of overlooking these concrete symptoms.

Also, in the formulation of single symptoms, I have been careful to see that the symptoms are actually representative of the proving, rather than just being there because they were found nowhere else in the Repertory. Making a single symptom is a risky business because it can be assumed, when one comes across it in the Repertory, as being unique only to that remedy, and found in no other. Whereas in many cases we know that the symptom may be present in another remedy, although it may not have been listed as the same/similar rubric. Despite all these safeguards, I do not deny that an element of subjectivity could have entered into these provings, and I doubt whether this could be altogether eliminated from any scientific observation.

This new method is still in an early stage and it is possible that it could have flaws, but the data, the actual experiences of the prover is invaluable information that can be used in practice, without restricting oneself to the viewpoint of the proving master. Taking a clue from one or two symptoms in a given case, the practitioner must examine the data from the actual provers, and it is possible that he might come to a startlingly different viewpoint than what had been summarized by the proving master.

The classification of remedies into kingdoms and the further realization of how closely connected the source of the substance is to the symptoms it produces, caused great enthusiasm, and a proliferation of theories and ideas on various substances. Some of these ideas were often more poetic than real, and were often backed by very incomplete or no provings. Through this book, I have attempted to demystify abstract ideas about substances, and instead represented provings as no more than collections of concrete data reported by the provers. While it must be admitted that there is a total connection between the remedy and its substance, often this connection is subtle, so that one cannot apply gross facts from the information abut the source and consider these as indications for the remedy. This is borne out by the earlier provings such as *Lac caninum*. If the reader reads through the proving very carefully and with circumspection, he may discover the spirit behind the substance.

1

THE PROVING OF *COCA-COLA*

The proving of *Coca-Cola* was conducted during my San Francisco seminar in May, 1994. The participants of the seminar were given one dose of the drug in the 30 C potency. They were instructed to note their symptoms over the next two days, whether they took the dose or not. The participants were not aware what substance was being proved. On the last day of the seminar, they gave up their notes. After these were read, we had a collective discussion of the symptomatology, and at the end of it, I told them the name of the remedy.

The drug was prepared at the Hahnemann Clinical Pharmacy, California, by Mr. Michael Quinn.

Note: The provers are here denoted by numbers. This proving being unsupervised and the group being large, it was difficult to know the provers on an individual basis. The symptoms that are reported here are taken directly from the notes that they had submitted to me. Since the symptoms were recorded over a period of only two days, and since many of the provers did not mention when the symptoms were experienced, information regarding the time of onset of the symptoms has not been included.

MIND

Emotions

Stoned / Spaced, etc.

- While walking, a sense of mellowness and extreme calm, both mental and physical; almost a sensation of anaesthesia of the body.

  [1/m/i]

- Felt drugged, as if my body had become very long, and I was falling fast through space. Later, felt introspectively "stoned" while talking.

  [23/m/i]

- Felt dull, as if I wasn't in touch with the others.

  [27/f/i]

- Feel light and happy, as if nothing matters much, and I can't control anything.

  [2'/f/S]

- Drank Coca-Cola so I could drive twelve hours through the night. It worked, but made me very sick. The room moved, as if I was being torn apart. It was the price I had to pay to get where I was going in time.

  [2'/f/S]

- "Mellow" feeling.

  [34/f/i]

- Felt "under the influence".

  [33/m/i]

- Feel my heart open to encompass all of humanity. Pleasant feeling of being expanded and boundless, not limited by the body.

  [11'/m/0]

Enjoyment / Amusement

- A sense of great pleasure in riding on trains and driving in all the hustle-bustle of city traffic. Confusion and giddiness at seeing people coming up and down elevators; it seemed as if no one knew where they were going. I found it amusing because if one were to get upset about it, it wouldn't make a difference.

  [22/f/i]

- Calm, enjoyment, great excitement and a sense of fun in the hustle-bustle in which I am usually uneasy and fearful to be alone.

  [28'/m/0]

- Desire to be amused by what I saw.

  [22/f/i]

- Giggling at seeing the confusion around.

  [25'/f/0]

Excitement

- Excited, nervous. Wanted to be social, have lively conversations, laugh.

  [2'/f/S]

- Cheerful, excited, talking fast.

  [33/m/i]

- An overwhelming rush, like after a steroid shot, "Go! Go! Go!"

  [4/f/i]

- Excitement, nervousness ameliorated from alcohol. Did not feel the usual hangover after alcohol.

  [4/f/i]

- Excited, and had an impulse to ride on cable cars.

[4/f/before dose]

- Very excited. Lots of energy.

[38/m/i]

Activity / Restlessness / Hurry

- Mind active and restless during sleep. Dreams all night.

[2'/f/S]

- Restless and agitated. A feeling of being tired, yet unable to sleep till late. Anxious about little things.

[6/f/i]

- Activity in the mind; wired and speedy.

[22/f/i]

- Mind overactive, busy, as in some sort of panic situation.

[43/f/i]

- Hurry, followed by tiredness.

[17/f/i]

- Hurried in eating.

[32/m/i]

- Irritable at the slow pace of the day.

[33/m/i]

- Mind very active at night, a halfway state between sleep and waking. Creative analogical thinking, of seeing relationships of desperate, seemingly discrete elements, pictorially juxtaposed, then a flash of intuition and new ideas emerging out of seemingly meaningless juxtapositions.

[50'/f/0]

Anxiety / Fear / Panic

- Very upset, nervous and frightened on realizing that I had made a mistake in the accounts. Fear that there won't be enough money. Cursed at husband when he asked me to calm down. Wondered how I could make this kind of mistake, being an accountant!

[2'/f/S]

- Feel frightened, everything looks strange. Miss roads I'm familiar with, and fear that I'll miss them again.

[2'/f/S]

- Fear that if I woke up in the middle of the night, I would not be able to return to sleep.

[4/f/i]

- Tense and anxious in the morning.

[15/*/i]

- Anxiety about being in time for the next day's appointment.

[19/*/i]

- Anxiety better in open air.

[25'/f/0]

- Panicky and hot at 1 a.m., after having realized that I would be in trouble for having forgtten something. Weeping, fear to be alone, fear of meeting an accident while driving. Was a complete wreck, the next morning.

[25'/f/0]

- Jumpy, nervous, but happy.

[2'/f/S]

Miscellaneous

- No strong emotion when my acquaintance jumped the queue on being recognized by the attendant in charge, and went ahead of me. It was as if I was only an observer.

[5/m/i]

- Slightly forgetful, but not worried about it.

[8'/f/0]

- Very social, more than usual.

[28'/m/0]

- Not sociable like I usually am.

[8'/f/0]

- Jolting out of sleep as from a shot in the head.

[38/m/i]

- Emotions flicker rapidly from happy, to frightened, to angry.

[2'/f/S]

- Feel scattered, as if thoughts not covered. Can't gather myself; need to depend on others.
[35'/*/0]
- Very indecisive, unsure of myself whether I should go out and eat when I wasn't hungry, be in the company of frenetic people who wanted to go dancing, to spend money.
[32/m/before remedy]
- Feel I will make a mistake; want someone else to tell me what to do.
[2'/f/S]
- Repeating counting rhymes from childhood in my mind, wondering if I have got them right.
[2'/f/S]
- Humming the song, "Somewhere over the Rainbow".
[7/f/i]
- Tormented by music. Unless I gave in and listened only to music, I felt tense and harassed by it.
[3/f/i]

- Annoyance from music, it had to be soft.
[25'/f/0]
- Rode on the wrong train, and then disappointed in myself for making such a stupid mistake; felt like crying.
[3/f/i]
- Feeling of sadness in the morning about life being so hard.
[42/f/i]
- Woke up with the sense of having a deep, deadly disease.
[15/*/i]
- Felt the need to become aware of my breathing – "Don't forget to breathe."
[35'/*/0]
- Irritable, critical and confrontational over nothing.
[49'/f/0]
- Started to feel the floor moving, undulating, disorienting under my feet. Almost fell because of this.
[50'/f/0]

Intellect

- Clarity of mind – could resolve several issues.
[1/m/i]
- Increased clarity of mind, despite lack of sleep.
[24/m/i]
- Unusually alert and then wondering for a moment where I was.
[37/f/i]
- Alertness combined with brief periods of exhaustion, tiredness and "flatness".
[4/f/i]
- Forgetful of a phone number I knew very well, and which I had remembered correctly only three hours ago.
[35'/*/0]

- Unable to remember things; feel foolish.
[2'/f/S]
- Losing her way in well-known streets.
[44/f/i]
- Got lost going home; went around and around.
[49'/f/0]
- Familiar streets looked unfamiliar, took the wrong way several times before finally coming onto the freeway.
[2'/f/S]
- Confusion, taking several wrong turns on streets and feeling lost.
[22/f/i]

- Started to feel different from my usual balanced self, and lost my orientation in traffic in a familiar area.
[24/m/i]

- Confused, lost, indecisive.
[25'/f/0]

- Dull and stupified in the afternoon.
[27/f/i]

- Confusion while doing a very simple lace pattern. Had to undo it and start over several times.
[33/m/i]

- Endless thoughts during the day.
[33/m/i]

- Thoughts about red worms crawling together with very little dirt, compost store, and bait shop. Thought also that I had worms in my stomach.
[8'/f/0]

- Had the thought that my veins were dark and could feel them exploding at the ends, especially in the arms.
[8'/f/0]

DREAMS

Children

- A friend learned through a phone call that his child had been stopped by the police while driving, and had received several fines amounting to two thousand nine hundred dollars, including one for the possession of narcotics.
[9/f/i]

- While in her kitchen, a mother notices for the first time that her son is an alcoholic, by seeing the large number of whisky bottle corks that he has collected. The corks have been perforated and arranged on strings in rows, like an abacus.
[10/m/i]

- I was telling my children, not to eat food they know will cause reactions. My friend's children were eating food that their mother had told them would cause itching. I commented that my children had been instructed to refuse such foods.
[3/f/i]

- I was dropping my son's friend back home and my son began to plead to be allowed to stay with his friend. I agreed. My mother and maternal grandmother (dead) were in front driving the car. As they pulled into the parking

lot, I wanted to go in and say hello to a woman I used to be involved with. My mother seemed unhappy with this, but agreed. As we were walking inside my son threw a rock which bounced up and hit a van. I warned him not to continue with such behaviour but he picked up another stone and a liquor bottle. I threatened him that he wouldn't be allowed to stay with his friend if he didn't put those down. He threw the stone which hit the other child on the head and began to run away. I became very angry and ran after him with the intention of catching him, pulling down his pants and spanking him. There were other children on the lawns, playing with liquor bottles.
[3/f/i]

- Three skinny, impoverished ragged children in the inner city. Eerie feeling, had to open my eyes to get the vision out of my mind.
[17/f/i]

- I walked over to reassure a retarded boy who was sitting, weeping, in a gutter outside his neighbours house, because he had been locked out, that his family would be home soon.
[26'/f/S]

Activity / Busy

- We are a huge crowd of ants running helter-shelter, like the bay to breakers race, only going all different ways.
  [2'/f/S]

- On a treasure hunt, keep changing the hide-out.
  [2'/f/S]

- Racing crowds.
  [2'/f/S]

- Moving up and down a tunnel but never quite finding the end.
  [30/m/i]

- A short man who was with me on a track was going to show me how to prepare to run a marathon.
  [33/m/i]

- Dreams of struggling all through the night.
  [38/m/i]

- Turbulent.
  [37/f/i]

- My cat chases and catches a large rat.
  [2'/f/S]

- Two cats chasing two mice, in my childhood home, but unable to catch them. We go from room to room and turn on the lights to help the cats. One mouse jumps into a waste basket and I try to trap it, but it crawls up my neck – was disgusted. It was an exciting but futile chase.
  [2'/f/S]

- On a wild ride in a car with an itchy, scaly man. Trying to get that man to the police and they didn't care much.
  [26'/f/S]

- Was trying to subdue a criminal, backstage, who had tried unsuccessfully to disturb a play, whose production crew I was a part of. I twisted his neck and strangled him without killing him. Later, I was in my child-hood home and the criminal was there. He had some medical monitor on his chest. I was running through a series of connecting rooms shouting that the police be called, afraid that he might harm my three-year old daughter or escape.
  [39/m/i]

- Several women following a blond girl across a stage, trying to imitate her eccentric motions as she teaches them classical Indian dance. The more she goes across the less she can remember until it all looks like clumsy karate chops.
  [2'/f/S]

- I was driving down a busy street with my boyfriend, at his suggestion that we should be in the car going somewhere rather than sleeping at home, when what I wanted to be doing was just that. He tried to take over the driver's seat. I got irritated and snap-ped at him saying that this was my car and I would do the driving. He was hurt, got out of the car and began to walk the way we came from. I was irritated that I had to deal with this, but realizing that I should get him back into the car, I turned round and convinced him to ride on the car, but insisted that we go back home and sleep some more.
  [3/f/i]

- I had moved the base of my operations because the company which I was working for had been sold. There had been a mishap and a new colleague of mine died in my pre-sence; I was unable to ressuscitate him with a special breathing pump that I had with me. I then went on a training mountaineering expedition with my new boss. It was very windy but warm, otherwise the conditions would have been severe. I awarded a grant of two billion dollars to a friend whose case I had agreed to take and who had been kind to me. I met with the Personnel Director of my new company and was concerned that they would not continue to keep me because of the incident of my colleague dying. There was a kind of whirlwind feeling of many events.
  [10/m/i]

■ I was on my way to a party at someone's house, and I was going through a maze of stores and restaurants. I remember one of the restaurants was the "Good Earth". In between the stores and restaurants instead of streets there were hallways.

I climbed a series of stairs to get to the house. It was on top of all the stores! I had to go to the top floor to convince two teenage boys to get ready for the party. One of them was wearing pyjamas that had belonged to my son when he was an infant. This boy was bouncing up and down on top of his bed, while the other was sitting down on his. I couldn't seem to get them moving to get dressed for the party. There seemed to be a lot of activity and confusion as to what was going on.

[44/f/i]

■ I was in a huge house, and was showing a Caucasian family around. They had two kids with them. The scene was quite busy. The woman had wandered off into one of the rooms. Someone found her there half naked, her clothes seeming like they had been torn off her body. She was smeared with chocolate all over, and was licking it off her fingers. She was on the floor, writhing in sensory ecstacy. A few of us tried to get her covered up and cleaned, but she was hard to grab, being in an agitated, intoxicated and insanely erotic state. As we tried to get the chocolate off her, it was getting smeared all over the carpet, and I was frantically trying to get the chocolate off the carpet. I was certain that the owner of the house would be very upset if I couldn't get it off. I woke up in the midst of that panic.

[44/f/i]

■ I am walking with my dogs. They are small, and ahead we see a huge black and white dog that looks like a cow. It charges at and chases the smaller ones. I am afraid that the dogs and me will be hurt, and I grab the big dog, call the others, and run into a building.

I panic, am breathing hard, my heart is pounding.

Then I have a container like a turtle aquarium with tiny dogs, greyhounds of two inches. One of them is white, and I think that they look like crickets rather than dogs. They keep hopping out, and I keep putting them back inside.

[48'/f/0]

Panic / Fear

■ No taxi driver is willing to take my wife and me home. One reluctantly agrees, and he begins to start the cab after I get in but my wife has still not boarded. I ask him to stop and he slows down, but again begins to move before she can get in. I panic; he has gone much ahead. I am asking him to stop. I get the feeling as if I am trying to control this driver, but he isn't coming under control, and I am wondering how to do it.

[43/f/i]

■ I was driving the car on the left side of a wet road, at night, in San Francisco. Suddenly there were no brakes, and the car continued to go downhill till it was out of control. I felt I should let down the bucket seat and lie flat so that I would prevent damage to myself in case some of the windows broke. But I felt there wasn't enough time to do that, and that I would hit something before I had the chance to ressuscitate myself.

The car began to spin around, having reached the bottom of the hill. I was amazed I hadn't crashed or hurt myself. Woke up breathing hard.

[7/f/i]

■ I was on the shores of an island, yelling to the others who had been stranded with me, to come back. They were attempting to wade or swim across very muddy, turbulent waters to the mainland very far away. A boat with some "bad men" was circling the island looking for one of the people, and I knew that we would all be in trouble if that person was found on the island. Felt anxious fearful and helpless.

[18'/f/0]

- Someone had entered my room in pitch darkness. I was terrified, wanted to move and get my knife, but was totally paralysed.

[36'/f/0]

- Terror.

[36'/f/0]

- I am seeing an old client in my office. I notice that the chairs, table, sofa and telephone are demolished. The closer I look, the more I see that it is demolished, and I wonder why I did not see it earlier. I panic.

[45/m/i]

Unconcerned / Calm

- Unconcerned, though I saw the police drive up while I was sitting on the side of highway, rolling a joint of marijuana. Felt no sense of anxiety; simply realized that I will have to eat the marijuana.

[1/m/i]

- Very calm and at ease with everyone at a college and high school reunion.

[27/f/i]

- Of not being upset on seeing a stainless steel pot with burn marks on it (normally would have been irritated).

[27/f/i]

- I had left my jacket, keys and wallet inside a van that had been set up as a museum. As I turned to go back to it, it started to drive away, and I calmly ran after it, following it, but lost it around the corner. A movie star came out from an apartment complex at the end of the road, greeted me and returned inside. I wondered how she knew me. I then mailed some letters a friend had given me to post. After this, my wife came to get me. I was not worried at all about getting home.

[27/f/i]

- I am invincible; there is a green aura around me to protect me. Someone with a samurai sword starts to stab me, but the sword is stopped by the green aura. I am invincible, totally whole, perfect, and one with myself – mind and body.

[46/m/i]

- The case I was to present at a course was incomplete. I realized I was going to die in two days, and was doing a last minute preparation. I was not upset, and was doing last minute jobs to clean things up. I was puzzled by two people who were concerned about my not being buried six feet under. (I was to be cremated, and placed at the threshold of the cremating gate just ten inches under.) This seemed like a silly concern on their part.

While doing all the day-to-day things, I thought surely there could be more interesting or more useful things to do, rather than daily drudgedy.

[47/f/i]

- Tall, powerful, black woman getting into a bar room brawl. Peaceful, distanced feeling.

[42/f/i]

Sexuality

- A beautiful, dark, slender, young man with soft, curly hair; delicate, gorgeous, feminine.

[2'/f/S]

- Female genitals that are enlarged, and starting to look like male genitals.

[2'/f/S]

- I was in the gym with a friend when a big, macho man came over and was being quite obnoxious. I told him he had a small penis, and that put him in his place. Then I was suddenly prompted to do many push-ups, even with one hand. I was sweating hard and breathing fast, with accelerated pulse rate – a feeling of omnipotence and power as though I was more male, though I felt powerful as a female.

[4/f/i]

- I was bored, listening to author Ronald Dahl complain about his difficulties with money, age, lack of freedom, etc., when I was transported into a new place dressed as a Las Vegas showgirl. I was accompanied by a similarly dressed girl, and we were being led by a man. We could only see his back and hear his voice. We were taken though a stage set which was a very large cavern, possibly in an underground area with blues, shimmering and sparkling lights. I realized that we were in a nest. The man sat down; he was costumed like a spider and around him was an enormous spider web with hand holds.

Then I realized that the woman and myself were "flies" and there was some cat and mouse game to be played. Instead of killing us when he caught us, he was going to have sex with us. I felt trapped, but also excited to play such an unusual game.

[4/f/i]

- Amorous.

[30/m/i]

- Making romantic gestures with an attractive woman in a movie theatre, when I realize it is not appropriate, she being my patient. I stop it kindly; I want all my patients to know that they are safe with me.

[42/f/i]

- Seeing photos of my wife and myself bathing, which I find quite erotic, while looking through a photo-album.

[1/m/i]

- I was in a multi-storeyed house that was so huge that it occupied a block. I had three sisters and a brother, and there were also some other people in the house. Two of the rooms in the upper right corner of the house were filled with very sensuous, sexual energy. I found myself in one of these rooms kissing my brother. I was getting ready to take off my clothes, when I opened my eyes and saw one of my sisters in the room. I tried to explain to her that I didn't know what was

happening; the sexual impulse had been just too strong to resist. She left the room in a hurry, and it was apparent that she had told everyone else, when later they all looked at me with disgust. I was at a loss as to what to do.

[44/f/i]

Wrong / Mistake

- Upset on finding that I had made a mistake.

[2'/f/S]

- Feeling guilty, as if I had committed a crime while taking the Princess out to a friend's. Felt like hiding the fact that I was taking her out, and then felt like I had done something wrong when the King and Queen "caught" me leaving. Also had the feeling that the King and Queen were not real, putting on a facade, not comfortable in their role.

[32/m/i]

- I am being told that my mother has uterine carcinoma and is very upset. I am busy, and forget to call her. I go home and find her very upset. I feel upset and guilty for not having called sooner. I feel like I did the wrong thing. I wonder what will I do about treating her cancer.

[48'/f/0]

- A friend who is like a father figure was watching a movie in a theatre with some other people. He stopped the movie with a remote controlled device to advise me that I shouldn't have had sex without having known her well. I was standing at the exit door in front of the theatre and it seemed as if I had made a mistake in getting involved with this woman and was in some kind of trouble for it.

[5/m/i]

- War, in which a pilot had been shot down. He was attacked by people, but apparently he had not done what they accused him of; in fact he was a hero.

[47/f/i]

- My son was to be kicked out of school

for something someone else had done. A theme of unfairness emerged, yet while explaining what had happened, my son told how he rode a bike over the sidewalk, and later lied to cover it up.

[47/f/i]

Floating

■ I was floating around the room in my home in Ireland, although my feet were on the ground. I could see all my family, yet it seemed that no one saw me.

[6/f/i]

■ I was floating through my school without anyone being aware of it. When I looked directly at my teacher's face it transformed into a devil's head with horns. When I looked away, it reverted back to her own head again, but as I again looked at her directly the same thing occurred. Felt strange, but not frightened.

[5/f/i]

■ Am observing myself during sleep, and lift myself out of sleep through levels of consciousness to the surface where I awaken.

[11'/m/0]

Miscellaneous

■ Easily climbing a chainlink fence, twenty feet high to retrieve a piece of paper that had been blownout of someone's hand.

[38/m/i]

■ Distributing food to stunned and unhappy looking Japanese people, who had been rounded up and placed in internment camps. Felt saddened by their plight and wanted to take care of them in the midst of their injustice. A year later, I once again strayed into such a centre in San Francisco in an area that was fenced off, and my wife and many young people came through the gate to join me.

[23/m/i]

■ Very unusually calmly helping a person in front of me who was unable to put a key into a lock by putting my hand over hers and gently guiding the key in.

[27/f/i]

■ Three men were trying to kill one man in an alley. I felt the need to go and help him.

[49/f/i]

■ I was to attend a teaching seminar in a place that looked like a school or monastery, but went downtown with a few others to save someone. There were two other friends there to help us and together we got this person out. We wanted to head back, but a truck which contained our possessions was parked on the street surrounded by hawkers and homeless street people. I grabbed a rectangular box which had some precious metal objects in it. Then a hooker came up to me and tried to seduce me, but I told her she could have the rest of the stuff in the truck (which she wanted anyway). Back in the monastery, I was in a room with another person when a large, kangaroo-like animal tried to get in through a hole in the screen. I was frightened and yelled to the other person to close the door. I could see the animal lying lengthwise against the building, as if I was looking through glass. Another animal with a white head got in through a hole in the wall, and though I was frightened at first, I later noticed it to be friendly and like a small, docile pig. Later, I had to go downstairs into the group area or kitchen of the monastery to get some keys, which I managed to grab after contorting my body around and down near the floor. Outside there were two or three homeless men near the loading dock. I began to speak to one of them who was friendly, but a little bit intoxicated and invasive of my space. I got back inside to see a monk verbally harassing a nun. She was upset and trying to go away, when he hugged her and threw her around gently, in fun. There was also a giant man who was surprised when another man he had been wrestling around with, flipped him so that he fell over a short wall and onto a table, on his back.

[15/∗/i]

▪ I had gone to a restaurant for breakfast with friends. We had to walk through the kitchen to be seated. The cooking area served as a counter for assorted electric griddles, frying pans, waffle makers, poachers, etc. There was an octopus of electric cords. Some stupid rednecks were staring at us.

I asked for juice, and the waitress brought us an imitation, artificial fruit drink. We asked for something real, and she brought us a beautiful, delicious, red-coloured juice made from pinenuts (which I dislike). There was a lot of plastic. I wondered how one can make something wonderful out of something "yucky". I felt the people were strange and backward. Also felt that the world was too chemical and synthetic; we were in a country where the food should be real, yet it is synthetic. I wondered what the world is coming to, and felt that the earth is going to be lost if we don't change our behaviour.

[40/m/i]

▪ I saw a cautioning sign while driving by a cove of water in an industrial setting, which warned that swimming there would cause suicidal feelings. Felt alone, melancholic, as if the world was sad and dark, and it was all madness.

[14/m/i]

▪ I was demonstrating to a woman the operation of a machine which had fluid flowing through tubes in its upper part and the controls in a lower part underneath. She seemed very pleased with how simple this made the task for her. Then when the woman was alone watching the operation and I was below turning some control, I heard her scream and knew she had been very badly injured. Some kind of acidic fluid had shot out of a tube that hadn't been properly connected, and I assumed that it had struck her eyes and possibly blinded her. I was in a

state of complete shock and despair.

[9/f/i]

▪ Quick, sudden, shocking, and startling dream of being struck in the groin with a blade-like knife, and ripped up through the head.

[6/f/i]

▪ I am the head in a house which is made of dirt, and get my grown son moving to work hard with me and accomplish a job that will help us to grow.

[19/∗/i]

▪ Being unable to fix the motor boat I was asked to.

[16'/m/0]

▪ My wife and I were looking for a place to stay on an island. We saw a sandy, narrow road around a cliff overlooking the ocean, which we could not consider since it would be impossible to drive a car on it. We saw one place that looked like a hotel, with prices for rooms on a sign outside.

[15/m/i]

▪ Finding a clean pot to urinate in inside a soiled public toilet into which I had walked barefoot.

[26/f/S]

▪ A father bought his pubertal aged sons a guitar that they were happily strumming in a music shop. They noticed street musicians in warm clothes, sitting on a blanket outside the shop, one of whom was playing a clarinet. Felt a magical feeling during the dream.

[10/m/i]

▪ Someone told me about a wonderful mountain they had been to and, on asking directions, they said they had walked on a peninsula that led to an ocean that led to the mountain.

[42/f/i]

▪ I had the idea to shoot someone, and was glad to see that the two guns that had been kept wrapped in brown paper in the trunk of my car had bullets. (Awoke panting, breathing fast.)

[14/m/i]

- I am standing in a field, and looking up at large pine trees. The sky is purplish of sureal colours, windy and stormy. The wind then kicks up and the sky is full of pine needles raining down. It's exciting and strange. A wild looking man with crazy eyes and a large mandible appears with an axe and begins to cut down a dead pine tree near him. People around him start yelling not to cut it because it could hurt someone if it falls onto the street.

[4/f/i]

- Some boys were trying to take away rabbits that a girl had hunted. It seemed as if they would succeed and she would lose her rabbits.

[2'/f/S]

- I was being evaluated by two famous homoeopaths for a remedy. The scene shifted, and I was witnessing a competition between chiropractors and homoeopaths. I wondered about the fairness of the competition.

[47/f/i]

- I was trying to get volunteers from the audience to continue a dance performance after the main entertainer had abruptly left to go to dinner. Someone asked me to volunteer, but I refused saying I had no particular entertainment skills. Then I announced someone from the audience I knew to be a good performer and he eagerly bounded up onto the stage, very happy to have had the opportunity to entertain.

[9/f/i]

- I was talking to someone on a street in Boston about wanting to do a duet piano recital with him at the conservatory. When he wondered who would come to hear, I replied we could do it for friends, family and ourselves.

Then I met my lawyer whom I hadn't met in a long time. He said he had been wanting to meet me. Another lawyer acquaintance put the ridiculous condition that the meeting needed to be in Spanish. I was angry and said that though I had wanted to learn Spanish, I was still an English speaker. The third person looked cheap and tacky, was wearing a blazer with a rip in the right shoulder seam and was flashing a big, insincere grin.

[3/f/i]

- I was gracefully descending a mountain to get into a cave. One or two friends accompanying me, who were above on the mountain, were worried that I would not be able to descend with my injured leg, but I did fine.

[3/f/i]

- I was joining group practice with another homoeopath and sharing a consulting room with her. The room was comfortable to be in and I wanted to spend time there. I offered to cover for her on some days and suggested that perhaps we could share coverage. I felt eager to please, ingratiating. She expressed concern about how I would care for her patients. She did not want me to vaccinate children too early or too much, and was also worried that I might prescribe allopathic medicine to her patients. I felt humbled, perhaps humiliated, but assured her I would not.

[3/f/i]

- A woman got into the bed with me and took up room. I felt crowded upon, and later on in the dream told a friend that the proving had something to do with boundaries.

[13'/m/0]

- I was on a bare dirt slope and had to go to work on some schedule and the others didn't. I went back to my home, and the man I had known twenty years ago as being pleasant but ignoring emotional issues, was there with some other people. They were rifling through food and had spilled granola on the floor of my old refrigerator. I felt intruded upon, and thought they were being insensitive and inconsiderate. I felt that I did not like this man any better than I used to.

[13'/m/0]

▪ A group of women consisting of my relatives were making rules for an organization. They had deliberately left out my cousin and me while voting. I stormed into the meeting angrily, and railed at them for their wrong and improper action. I sorted through a mess of bits and pieces of paper with the help of my daughter to find the womens' by-laws that talk about this behaviour. As I stormed out, slamming the door, I heard my grandmother say under her breath that I hound her.

[38/m/i]

▪ I was walking across in the street in a cold, desolate area of town I call "no man's land". It was isolated. I wanted to buy something, perhaps lunch, but no stores were open. It was a very bleak feeling.

[3/f/i]

▪ I was living in a small, dirty, bare mountain cottage. It was Christmas eve and there were some dogs there that I liked but which did not belong to me. Then I was in a large bar that was bare with only a few people in it. Oddly, I saw a woman I knew, with her partner and child. It was cold and bare outside and inside as well, the room was big, hollow and resounding, and bare of any warmth and festivity. A bar-tender was serving us and there was an older, stocky man who decided to leave, although there was some rule against leaving early. He was telling to the bar-tender in a surly, contentious way he would do what he wanted. I asked him how he got to leave and he said that he was with the CIA and had just shown the bar-tender a small, silvery knife issued by the CIA.

After a while we all left to go home for the rest of Christmas.

[13'/m/0]

▪ Called on a friend who was happy to see me, and then showed me his sore throat. I was disappointed that it was the doctor he had wanted to see.

[42/f/i]

▪ I have been captured and about to be sent to a prison camp while doing a dangerous job as an agent for the resistance in a fascist state in Europe. A woman is standing over me and psychologically intimidating me. I must acquiesce, or suffer some kind of humiliation and/or punishment. I am made to watch the search of girl child of five or six years of age as she is being humiliated and slapped around by the woman. A knife has been confiscated from the child and a blade recovered after slashing open the collar of her woolen sweater. The "bitch" tells me that the child is only seventeen months old and has been working like that for four months. She glares at me, as if expecting some kind of response. My heart goes out to the brave little girl, yet I am terrified. I cast my eyes down and murmur that she is brave.

Then I notice a raw, red, wet, oozing eczema behind one of the girl's knees, and I have the recollection of having treated her in the past. I advise the "bitch", who now appears like a mother figure to her, to wash the rash daily with diluted vinegar. When she says she has tried it before, I tell her she needs to be persistent and should go to a health store to buy rice wine vinegar, and dilute it just enough so that it doesn't sting on application. She makes notes in gold ink in a crowded organizer on a much written page.

[3/f/i]

▪ Deciding between being with old friends who are off to see a space needle, and being with my wife and children whom I am vacationing with and who will feel sad to have me gone.

[23/m/i]

- Giardia lambdia.

[10/m/i]

- A young lady friend who was waiting in a queue with me commented that I was so mild and smiled a lot. I agreed and replied that I would brood. I was making faces to her and then laughed.

[31'/f/0]

- Orange colour.

[34/f/i]

- Reunion with family and class.

[34/f/i]

- Husband cutting his hair.

[2'/f/S]

- I toss back a basketball that has bounced through the window of my bedroom in my childhood home, from a game being played between rowdy menacing teenage boys below.

[10/m/i]

- Vivid, coloured dreams.

[11'/m/0]

- Wandering through a park looking for a particular building, while the person accompanying me goes off to find something.

[11/m/0]

- Grave situation where a sick, blond haired, model-like woman was lying in a cot, perhaps near death.

[10/m/i]

- An old couple who loved each other very much sitting on a park bench. They did not want to travel anywhere to get the care they needed.

[37/f/i]

- Michael Jackson.

[21/f/i]

- My wife was in a bathtub in a large place that looked like a village. I fell in with my glasses on, while I waited for her.

[39/m/i]

- Going to a pot luck.

[40/m/i]

- Police arriving where a car had run into trouble or had an accident.

[40/m/i]

- I have gone back to medical school with the feeling that I hadn't learned enough. I take an essay test and am unhappy at my low scores. I try to talk gently to a woman teacher about two questions that were unclear, but she becomes defensive and accuses me of personality flaws.

Then I am in a lecture room, and a patient of mine is seated behind me, and is eating carrots out of my plate in a rather affectionate way. I am nervous because I do not want people to get the idea that we are romantically involved. She seems interested in me and I do not want her to be hurt by people's view of herself, but I can't say anything or it will make it more obvious.

Then a Persian first year student with a tendency to party and ballroom dance, but who is buckling down to work, asks me kindly why I have come back to medical school when others think I am a great doctor who has helped many people. I realize I had been happier practising, and consider quitting school and resuming practice. I feel lost; I am not doing what I am supposed to.

[42/f/i]

- Ocean crashing down on streets.

[30/m/i]

- A woman with purplish hair was walking softly, bare-footed on the deck of a ferryboat so as not to disturb the people below her. She was later explaining how boats come up during a storm. She narrated one occasion where the water rose and pushed her bed up into the ceiling of the boat, and her corral pieces got crushed on the ceiling.

[42/f/i]

- Outdoors, swimming-pool.

[42/f/i]

- An ex-lover visited me to tell me that he was going to pick me up on Saturday night. He was not asking to pick me up, rather was telling me. I tried to explain that I couldn't or wouldn't, and so forth, but was unable to get a word in. He just kept repeating the announcement that he was going to pick me up on Saturday night and that was the end of the story. He wouldn't listen to anything I had to say.

[44/f/i]

STRANGE PHENOMENA DURING PROVING

- The alarm that I had set at 6.00 a.m. moved ahead twice to 8.30, in spite of careful checking.

[13'/m/0]

- Saw three homeless people with dyed hair cut in punk hairdos, wearing oversized rags for clothes, and with their heads bowed low. They huddled together for warmth and security as if they were in a jungle of fear and isolation. I thought it was as if someone had sold them a train ticket that was advertised to take them to a great place. They had got on the train and realized that the place they got to is horrible, lonely and desperate, but they didn't know how to leave or how to change their reality; it was sad. I thought the movie, "The Gods Must Be Crazy" epitomises the whole situation. First, there is peace and harmony, then the coke bottle drops down and the craziness starts; violence, anger, jealousy, irrationality.

[22/f/i]

- Drank Coca-Cola for the first time in years. Wondered why I was drinking this, I didn't like this taste.

[37/f/i]

- Expressed surprise that a colleague drank Pepsi-Cola, and then said, with a kind of serious and sleepy dismay, that Coca-Cola was what was wrong with the whole world, and that we had exported it all over the world. Then paused and asked my colleague if she understood this symbolic, rather drastic statement.

[41/f/0]

PHYSICAL SYMPTOMS

Generalities

- Sensitive to touch, uncomfortable from pressure.

[2'/f/S]

- Feel cold to the bone from wind.

[8'/f/0]

- Very tired, with decreased appetite and thirst.

[12/*/i]

- Tiredness on waking in the morning.

[13'/m/0]

- Tiredness.

[17/f/i]

- Tightness in the body from panic.
  [25'/f/0]
- Desire for sweets.
  [32/m/i]
- Desire for bread.
  [33/m/i]
- Exhaustion between 9.00-10.00 a.m. and 2.00-9.00 p.m.
  [35'/*/0]

- Chilly; desire for warm clothing.
  [35'/*/0]
- Was able to tolerate ice-water that I usually hate.
  [42/f/i]
- Desires tea.
  [49'/f/0]

Particular symptoms

Head
- Dull ache in temples, left side, worse than right.
  [3/f/i]
- Pleasant vibration felt strongly in head.
  [11'/m/0]
- Tension in occiput.
  [15/*/i]
- Light headed with panic.
  [25'/f/0]
- Mild pain over eyebrows.
  [30/m/i]
- Pain – left side.
  [37/f/i]
- Old intermediate, chronic headache in both temples, as of a vice, reappeared at night and was gone in the morning.
  [42/f/i]

Ears and hearing
- Ringing in the left ear.
  [8'/f/0]

Nose
- Nasal congestion.
  [3/f/i]
- Fullness of sinuses, clearing at times.
  [4/f/i]
- Sneezing, which ameliorated; felt peaceful, clear in the sinuses, as after doing Pranayama.
  [5/m/i]

Face
- Tension in jaw.
  [15/*/i]
- Eruptions on left cheek.
  [33/m/i]

Mouth and taste
- Taste bitter for sweet raisins.
  [2'/f/S]
- Dryness.
  [4/f/i]
- Tapping teeth together.
  [5/m/i]
- Dryness, on waking from frightful dream.
  [7/f/i]
- Salivation on waking. Tongue felt an odd shape.
  [14'/m/0]

Throat
- Heartburn.
  [2'/f/S]
- Congestion, raw pain and swollen sensation from throat to ears.
  [3/f/i]

---

1 Yogic exercise; form of meditation through the regulation of breath.

Stomach

- Nausea from Coca-Cola.

[2'/f/S]

- Burning in stomach.

[2'/f/S]

- Strange, uneasy sensation, a queeziness, a hollow, empty feeling like a vibrating violin string after listening to some strange, unmelodic, repetitive music. Aggravated in the evening.

[3/f/S]

- Gurgling and cramps in the stomach with hunger.

[8'/f/0]

- Eructations.

[8'/f/0]

- Eructations.

[12/*/i]

- Have to hold and rub stomach.

[12/*/i]

- Nausea with panic.

[12/*/i]

- Tingling sensation in solar plexus.

[27/f/i]

- Increased appetite.

[4/f/i]

- Feeling very hungry.

[8/f/0]

Abdomen

- Pain in bowels and increased flatulence.

[4/f/i]

- Gurgling, incarcerated flatus.

[10/m/i]

Rectum and stool

- Diarrhoea from Coca-Cola.

[2'/f/S]

- Slight diarrhoea on waking in the morning. Large amounts of soft stool at night with cramping in abdomen and a lot of gas.

[8'/f/0]

- Sputtering diarrhoea.

[10/m/i]

- Liquid, yellow-brown diarrhoea between 3.00 a.m.-5.00 a.m.

[12/*/i]

- Painless diarrhoea.

[13'/m/]

- Severe foul smelling diarrhoea with flatus.

[25/f/0]

- Urge to stool from anticipatory anxiety.

[28'/m/0]

- Diarrhoea, watery.

[48/f/i]

Urinary organs

- Desire to urinate at night.

[26'/f/S]

Respiration

- Lungs aching from breathing very hard during frightful dream.

[7/f/i]

- Panting, breathing fast on waking.

[14/m/i]

Chest

- Rash on chest.

[2'/f/S]

Back

- Pleasant vibration in back.

[11'/m/0]

- Pain in the tail bone, comes and goes gradually.

[31'/f/0]

- Sensation of heat going up my spine.

[32/m/i]

Extremities

- Sensation as of an electric shock in the fingers of the right hand.

[1/m/i]

- Heat of the hands.

[2'/f/S]

- Painful cramp in leg and fourth-fifth

metatarsal area of foot.

[5/m/i]

- Restless legs – wanted to stretch them all the time.

[6/f/i]

- Swelling and redness in right toe at night, with bruised pain as from a spike, in the inner aspect.

[8'/f/i]

- Numbness in left hand on waking.

[14/m/i]

- Mild cramping in right leg. Numbness in both legs like they are falling asleep.

[30/m/i]

- Coldness and numbness of hands.

[30/m/i]

- Coldness of hands, and around ankles.

[35'/*/i]

- Pain in wrists, especially left, at noon.

[42/f/i]

Sleep

- Refreshed and alert from shorter duration of sleep.

[4f/i]

- Disturbed between 7.00 a.m. and 8.00 a.m.

[7/f/i]

- Sleepiness, taking many short naps during the day.

[8'/f/0]

- Sleepiness during the day.

[11'/m/0]

- Drowsy during the day.

[13'/m/0]

- Arms and hands clenched over heart area during sleep.

[15/*/i]

- Unable to sleep till late, though tired.

[17/f/i]

- Waking at 5.00 a.m. with restlessness and inability to go back to sleep.

[18'/f/0]

- Restful sleep. Alert in spite of waking early.

[25'/f/0]

- Severe insomnia – mind was racing.

[25'/f/0]

- Sleeplessness.

[33/m/i]

- Yawning, sleepiness during day.

[35'/*/0]

- Deep sleep.

[37/f/i]

- Position – on left side.

[42/f/i]

Perspiration

- Profuse sweat which wet the quilt around.

[5/m/i]

Skin

- Itchy, skin very sensitive.

[2'/f/S]

RUBRICS

Mind

Single symptoms
- Activity, panic, as from.
- Alertness, alternating with confusion as to where she is.
- Alertness, alternating with exhaustion and dullness.
- Amusement, confusion and hustle-bustle, at.
- Anaesthesia, sensation of.
- Anxiety, time is set, if a, anxious about the next day's appointment.
- Clarity of mind, clear, everything seems, so that he can resolve all issues.
- Delusion, expanding and boundless, he is.
- Delusion, falling fast, space, through.
- Delusion, heart open, was, to encompass all humanity.
- Delusion, lost in a big city, as if.
- Delusion, scattered, she was, could not collect herself and had to depend on others.
- Delusion, torn apart, she was being.
- Dreams, accidents, operating machine, while.
- Dreams, animals, kangaroo-like.
- Dreams, animals, large.
- Dreams, animals, mouse, crawling up her neck.
- Dreams, animals, mouse trying to trap, a fleeing.
- Dreams, animals, pig.
- Dreams, animals, room, were trying to break into.
- Dreams, ants, his group was a.
- Dreams, bed, crowded, upon being.
- Dreams, body, body parts, knee, wet eczema.
- Dreams, bottles, of throwing.
- Dreams, boys, boy retarded, locked out of his house and weeping in a gutter.
- Dreams, boys, rowdy, menacing.
- Dreams, boys, trying to take away from a girl rabbits she had hunted.
- Dreams, building, looking for a particular.
- Dreams, car ride, he was on, wild.
- Dreams, cars, spinning, going out of control.
- Dreams, caught, of being.
- Dreams, caught for possessing narcotics.
- Dreams, cautioned, of being.
- Dreams, cautioning others, of.
- Dreams, children, alcoholic, her son was a.
- Dreams, children, control, her son, she was trying to.
- Dreams, children, liquor bottles, playing with.
- Dreams, climbing, high fence with ease.
- Dreams, confidence in her, her colleague did not have.
- Dreams, cottage, small, dirty, bare.
- Dreams, couple, old loving.
- Dreams, colour, orange.
- Dreams, criminal, running around.
- Dreams, criminal, trying to subdue a.
- Dreams, crowds, of racing.
- Dreams, dancing, following eccentric

dance steps.
— Dreams, driving down a busy street against her will.
— Dreams, eerie, skinny, impoverished, ragged looking children in the inner city.
— Dreams, electric wires, many.
— Dreams, events, many, whirlwind-like.
— Dreams, face, transformed into a devil's head with horns.
— Dreams, food, distributing in a war camp.
— Dreams, food, synthetic, of.
— Dreams, foreign language, she had to converse in.
— Dreams, games of, cat and mouse like.
— Dreams, games, of sex.
— Dreams, genitalia, female, enlarged like male genitals.
— Dreams, grant, of awarding a large.
— Dreams, guitar, of buying a.
— Dreams, haircut.
— Dreams, helping other people, of.
— Dreams, homeless men.
— Dreams, humiliation, of.
— Dreams, insect, she was a.
— Dreams, intoxicated persons, of.
— Dreams, intruded upon, she was being.
— Dreams, job, he would lose his.
— Dreams, knife, struck in the groin with a, and ripped up through the head.
— Dreams, lifted, she was, out of her body.
— Dreams, machine, demonstrating the operation of a.
— Dreams, magical.
— Dreams, man crazy, looking eyes, with.
— Dreams, man, feminine looking.
— Dreams, man, obnoxious, big macho.
— Dreams, mistakes, of.
— Dreams, mountain, descending, despite her injured leg.
— Dreams, mountaineering expedition, of.
— Dreams, notes, making, on a much written page.
— Dreams, panicky, that the taxi kept moving ahead each time his wife tried to get inside.
— Dreams, ocean crashing down on street.
— Dreams, paralysed, she was, fear from.
— Dream, peninsula, ocean and mountain, of.
— Dream, police, unconcernedly rolling a marijuana cigarette, in the presence of.
— Dream, pot luck, of going to.
— Dreams, powerful and male, of feeling (in a woman).
— Dream, pursuing, she helped cats chase mice.
— Dreams, revive, he was unable to, his dying friend.
— Dreams, romantic.
— Dreams, save someone, he had to.
— Dreams, searching for a place to stay on an island.
— Dreams, shooting.
— Dreams, sick, blond woman.
— Dreams, sky, purplish, surreal.
— Dreams, struggling, of.
— Dreams, teacher, accused her of personality flaws.
— Dreams, trapped.
— Dreams, treasure hunt, on a, the hideout kept changing.
— Dreams, trees being cut.
— Dreams, tunnel, he moved up and down a, but never found its end.
— Dreams, turbulent.

— Dreams, walking, alone in a isolated street.
— Dreams, war camp, of being in.
— Dreams, water, rising during a storm.
— Dreams, worms, round worms.
— Excitement, alcohol ameliorates.
— Fear, morning, waking on, disease, deadly, of.
— Fear, night, waking after.
— Giggling, confusion, all around her, at.
— Impatience, rush about, he must.
— Impulse, cable cars to ride.
— Irritability, slow pace of the day, at.
— Lightness and happiness, feeling of, as if nothing mattered, and she could not control anything.
— Music, agreeable, soft.
— Music, annoyance, from.
— Repeats, rhymes, childhood, from.
— Sadness, melancholy, hardships of life, about.
— Starting, sleep from, jolting as from a shot through the head.
— Thoughts, worms, about.
— Thoughts, veins were dark and exploding at the ends.
— Weeping, tearful mood, mistakes, over his.

Common symptoms
— *Activity, desires*.
— Amusement, desire for.
— *Anxiety*.
— Anxiety, morning.
— Anxiety, air, open ameliorates.
— Anxiety, trifles, about.
— Cheerfulness.
— Confidence, want of self.
— **Confusion of mind, loses his way in well-known streets.**

— Cursing, swearing, blasphemy, profanity.
— Delusion, body long, too.
— Delusion, strange, everything seems.
— Delusion, worms, creeping, of.
— Dreams, accidents.
— Dreams, amorous.
— Dreams, anxious.
— Dreams, animals, cat pursuing a mouse (*Ocimum sanctum*).
— Dreams, danger, of.
— Dreams, colourful.
— Dreams, dead relatives, of.
— Dreams, disgusting.
— Dreams, excrement, wading though.
— Dreams, floating.
— Dreams, movie star (Black mamba, *Lac leoninum*).
— Dreams, police.
— Dreams, unsuccessful efforts.
— Dreams, vivid.
— Excitement, excitable.
— Fear, accidents.
— Fear, mistakes.
— Fear, poverty.
— Helplessness, feeling of.
— High spirited.
— Hurry, haste.
— Hurry, haste, eating, while.
— Hurry, haste, fatigued, gets.
— Impulsive.
— Indifference, apathy.
— Indifference, apathy, complain, does not.
— Indifference, apathy, external things, to.
— Indifference, apathy, irritating, disagreeable things, to.
— Irresolution.
— Irresolution, laughing.

— Lightness, feeling of.
— **Mistakes, localities, in.**
— Moods, changeable, variable.
— Music aggravates.
— Prostration of mind, mental exhaustion, brain fag.
— Quick to act.
— *Restlessness, nervousness.*
— Restlessness, nervousness, sleeplessness, with.

— Reproaches himself.
— Sensitive, oversensitive, music, to.
— Singing, humming to herself.
— Stupefaction, as if intoxicated.
— Thoughts, rush, flow of, sleeplessness.
— Torpor.
— Tranquility, serenity, calmness
— Vivaciousness.

Physical symptoms

Generalities
— Cold, aggravates.
— Cold, feeling, bones.
— Food and drinks, bread, desire.
— Food and drinks, sweets, desire.
— Food and drinks, tea desire.
— Pressure aggravates.
— Touch aggravates.
— Sneezing ameliorates.
— Stiffness.
— Warm clothing, desire.
— Weariness.
— Weariness, morning, 9.00 a.m.-10.00 a.m.
— Weariness, morning, waking on.
— Weariness, afternoon, 2.00 p.m.-9.00 p.m.
— Wind.

Head
— Constriction, occiput.
— Lightness, sensation of, panic with (single).

— *Pain.*
— Pain, forehead, eyes above.
— Pain, sides, left.
— Pain, dull pain, temples.
— Pain, pressing, vise, as if in a.
— Pain, pressing, temples.
— Pain, pressing, temples, morning ameliorates (single).
— Pain, pressing, temples, night.
— Vibrations, sensation of, pleasant (single).

Ear
— Noises, ringing, left.

Nose
— Congestion, nose, to.
— Fullness, sense of.

Face
— Eruptions, cheek, left.
— Tension, jaw, lower.

Mouth
— Dryness.

- Dryness, night, waking on.
- Salivation, morning, waking on.
- Taste, bitter, sweet things taste, raisins (single).

Teeth

- Grinding.

Throat

- Fullness.
- Pain, burning.
- Pain, raw.
- Pain, raw, extending to ears.
- Swelling, sensation of.

Stomach

- Appetite, diminished.
- Appetite, increased.
- Emptiness.
- Emptiness, evening.
- Emptiness, music aggravates, hollow feeling like a vibrating violin string (single).
- Eructations.
- Gurgling.
- Heartburn.
- *Nausea.*
- Nausea, anxiety, with.
- Nausea, Coca-Cola, from (single).
- Pain, burning.
- Pain, cramping.
- Pain, cramping, hunger from (single).
- Rub, hold and rub stomach, must (single).
- Thirstless.
- Tingling.

Abdomen

- *Flatulence.*
- Flatulence, obstructed.

- Gurgling.
- Pain, cramping.

Rectum

- Diarrhoea.
- Diarrhoea, morning.
- Diarrhoea, midnight after 3.00-5.00 a.m. (single).
- Diarrhoea, Coca-Cola aggravates (single).
- Diarrhoea, painless.
- Flatus, stool during.
- Urging, anxious.

Stool

- Brown.
- Copious.
- Flatulent.
- Odour, offensive.
- Soft.
- Sputtering.
- Thin.
- Yellow.

Bladder

- Urging to urinate night.

Respiration

- Panting, waking, on.
- Accelerated, waking, on.

Cheese

- Eruptions, rash.
- Pain, lungs.

Back

- Heat, spine, extending upward.
- Pain, coccyx, appears gradually and disappears gradually (single).
- Vibration, sensation of, pleasant (single).

Extremities

- Coldness, hands.
- Coldness, ankles.
- Cramps, leg.
- Cramps, foot.
- Discolouration, redness, hand.
- Electrical current, sensation of, fingers, right hand (single).
- Heat, hand.
- Pain, upper limbs, wrist, left.
- Pain, upper limbs, wrist, afternoon.
- Pain, sore, bruised, toes.
- Pain, sore bruised, toes first, right (single).
- Pain, splinter, as if, first, right.
- Numbness, insensibility, hand, left.
- Numbness, insensibility, morning, waking on.
- Numbness, insensibility, leg.
- Numbness, insensibility, hand.
- Restlessness, legs, stretch legs, desire to.
- Swelling, toes, first, right.

Sleep

- Deep.
- Disturbed, morning, 7.00 a.m.-8.00 a.m., between (single).
- Falling asleep, difficult.
- Falling asleep, late.
- Position, arms, hands, heart area, clenched over (single).
- Position, side, on left.
- Restless.
- Short refreshes.
- Sleepiness.
- Sleepiness, daytime.
- Sleeplessness.
- Sleeplessness, morning 5.00 a.m., after.
- Sleeplessness, thoughts, from.
- Yawning, daytime.

Perspiration

- Profuse.
- Profuse, sleep, during.

Skin

- Itching.
- Sensitiveness.

THEMES

1. **Activity and excitement**

   Restless, nervous, hurried, jumpy.

   Social, lively.

   Agitation, overwhelming rush.

   Sleepless. Mind racing, busy, overactive.

   Wiry and speedy.

   Anxiety about being in time for the next days appointment.

   Lots of energy.

   Treasure hunt, the hideout kept changing.

   Cats chasing mice.

   Wild car ride.

   Racing crowds.

   Forced to drive in busy street.

   Dancing.

   Going up and down a tunnel without finding its end.

2. **Confusion**

   Making mistakes. Taking wrong turns.

   Losing his way in well-known streets.

   Indecisive.

   Scattered, thoughts.

   Ants running helter-skelter.

   Amusement, giggling, enjoyment at the hustle, bustle and confusion.

   Car going out of control.

   Taxi driver not coming under control.

   Children throwing stones, bottles.

   Children on narcotics, alcohol.

3. **The world was sad, it was all madness**

   The world is too chemical and synthetic. We will lose the world if we don't change.

   Craziness, violence, anger, jealousy, irrationality.

   ("The Gods Must be Crazy.")

4. **Tranquillity, calmness, anaesthesia, mellow feeling**

   Stoned. Drugged.

   Indifferent. Unconcerned, though in the possession of narcotics.

5. **Clarity of kind, despite lack of sleep**

6. Making a mistake.

   Everything looks strange.

   Accident while operating machine.

   House being broken into.

   Improverished, ragged, skinny, children, eerie looking.

   Losing his job.

7. **Change of emotions: "rapid flicker" from frightened to angry**

8. **Desolate area, "No man's land"**

   In a jungle of fear and isolation.

9. **Crowds**

   Bed crowded upon.

   Intrusive persons.

   Racing crowds.

10. **Anxiety for others**

    Helping others.

11. **Surreal colours, exciting**

    Wonderful mountain peninsula.

    Magical.

    Light and happy.

    Floating. Lighting through levels of consciousness.

12. **Old, loving couple**

13. **Thoughts**
    Worms.
    Compost.
    Veins exploding.

14. **Sexuality**
    A feminine looking man.

Female feeling more male and powerful.

Sex games: cat and mouse, spider and flies.

Erotic and amorous dreams.

15. **Disgusting dreams**

2

THE PROVING OF *CROTALUS CASCAVELLA*

I conducted a proving of *Crotalus cascavella* in April 1995. Twelve provers participated, none of whom knew what was being proved. The provers were between twenty-two to thirty years in age. They were given one dose each in the 30 C potency, and asked to note their symptoms. All of them took the dose except prover L. The provers met with me individually once a week and after three weeks they met as a group. During the meeting, the proving was discussed and the name of the substance revealed. Any further symptoms that were noted after the discussion of the proving were reported to the master prover, and have been incorporated into the proving.

The drug was obtained from the pharmacy "Roy and Company", Bombay.

MIND

Emotions

Alone

- I feel as if my friends share my joy with me, but am unsure whether they would share my sorrow. Felt that no one listens to me, as if my words are of no value, even though I care a lot for my friends. I felt God would help me so that one day they will realize my importance. Felt a sense of isolation.

[G/m/2,*/i]

- A constant fear and anxiety that I might make a mistake, or do something wrong in the future as a result of which my friends will not want me anymore. Fear that I will be left alone.

[H/f/1,*/i]

- Was unusually sympathetic towards a younger cousin whose parents were away. Felt she is all alone, has no one with her. Was careful not to hurt her.

[A/f/1,*/i]

- Feel like being alone during abdominal pain. Feel like going back home where I am safe.

[B/m/3,*/i]

Friends

- Insecure; do not like my friends talking to others. Feel they should talk only with me, and be only with me.

[G/m/1,*/i]

- Became very possessive about my best friends. Was sensitive to people making fun of them, to them going away from me.

[H/f/1,*/i]

- Felt like speaking with my friends very often.

[K/f/1,*/i]

- Mistrustful about friends; do not know whether the things they tell me are right or wrong.

[G/m/2,*/i]

Fears

- Woke up in the night with the feeling that I had heard a loud noise, like a cow's moo. Then felt it could be a ghost. Was afraid to go back to sleep, to switch off the lights, to shut the window. Felt it could be anywhere, and that it might come when I am off-guard and do something horrible to me. Later felt stupid for having been afraid.

[B/m/1,1/i]

- Did not want to be "hassled" anymore by beggars. Decided to get tough on them, to take action straight away. But was afraid that they might form a gang and attack and harm me when I was alone in the dark, or that they would not help me out in the event that I was attacked by someone else.

[B/m/2,*/i]

- Had the sensation, when alone, as if I was being followed. Looked around me several times.

[B/m/3,*/i]

- Waking between 2.30 and 3.00 a.m., to check that there had been no theft.
[F/m/1,*/i]

- Constantly checking to see if I am carrying my train pass, with a fear of being caught and the subsequent embarrassment.
[J/f/3,*/i]

- Startle at the slightest noise.
[L'/f/*,*/0]

- Felt a sense of injustice about men getting into the ladies compartment of a train. Complained about it to a policeman, but was afraid that they would follow me.
[J/f/2,*/i]

Anxiety

- Usual anxiety about the future was ameliorated. Felt calm, tension free, with a feeling that I would face the future as it came.
[A/f/1,*/i]

- Insecure, nervous about the future with palpitations.
[G/m/1,*/i]

- Tension – as when coming down a giant wheel.
[H/f/1,*/i]

- Show I am happy, although tense and insecure.
[G/m/*,*/i]

- Very much anxious for sister (who was depressed), panicked. Much concern for her. Tried to keep the environment light by telling her jokes, tried to divert her attention by taking her to movies and for long walks. Felt responsible for her.
[F/m/1,*/i]

Irritability / Anger

- Was irritated at a colleague for repeatedly questioning a patient. Felt he was "after him". Felt angry and irritated at the patient's lack of response. Got up and left in anger.
[D/f/1,1/i]

- Irritated; "on my nerves". Wanted to ask a colleague to "shut up and get lost". Couldn't stay in her presence, wanted to get up and leave.
[C/f/1,1/i]

- Anger, "burst out" at mother for asking what I thought was a "stupid question".
[C/f/1,1/i]

- Irritable at trifles.
[C/f/1,1/i]

- Was "wild" at my mother for not having listened to me. Would not listen to reason, was unmoved by apologies.
[D/f/3,*/i]

- Very irritable mood.
[G/m/1,*/i]

- Irritable at trifles; when things went against me; when I felt I was being forced to do something.
[H/f/1,*/i]

- Anger on contradiction; when not listened to.
[H/f/2,*/i]

- Anger increased when hungry.
[B/m/3,*/i]

- Irritated, did not want to talk with a physician who I felt was going off in a totally opposite direction while discussing a case. Wanted to get out of there.
[C/f/3,*/i]

- Anger at trifles, without knowing why.
[G/m/2,*/i]

- Started a discussion about men making passes at women in crowded places. Felt anger towards such men.
[A/f/3,*/i]

Violence

- Was angry at a colleague for being arrogant, for not letting me speak. Wanted to hit him, to throw him out.
[C/f/1,*/i]

- Enjoyed crushing mosquitoes and small cockroaches. Enjoyed violence, derived a sadistic pleasure from it.

[B/m/2,*/i]

- Very violent anger when things do not go the way I expect them to. As a result, people treat me with great care and respect. Want to "finish them off".

[B/m/2,*/i]

- Desire to violently attack, slit up others with a very sharp knife, when I feel attacked.

[B/m/3,*/i]

- Thoughts, only of killing.

[G/m/*,*/i]

- Felt a kind of madness where I wanted to kill anyone who disturbed me. But fearing punishment from God, thought that I would only teach them a lesson.

[G/m/*,*/i]

- Desire to slap someone if they tried something "funny" with me. Felt very angry at men who followed girls; felt they were "bastards", and should be shot point blank. But was unable to do anything for the fear of being raped.

[C/f/*,*/i]

- Was angry at a man who deliberately brushed against me. Shouted at him, caught him and hit him, and felt that all of his kind should be hit. Anger followed by loud, cause-less laughter.

[L'/f/*,*/0]

- Felt that eve-teasers should be stabbed, shooting was too easy for them. Wanted to do them physical harm, kill them. But was cautious in a public place, because I was afraid that they might come back and take revenge. I felt in such an eventuality, no one would come to my rescue; I would have to fight for myself, would be helpless.

[L'/f/*,*/0]

- Angry, towards eve-teasers; wanted to hit them, to harm them, to make them realize how it feels, by something similar happening to one of their family.

[K/f/*,*/i]

Two wills

- A feeling of being tremendously exploited by my landlords; I felt that they were taking maximum advantage without giving me anything in return. Was angry; felt violent, near explosion. Wanted to destroy, smash up the building, set it on fire; could not hold it anymore. On the other hand, knew that I could not do it because it was illegal, and I would get into trouble with the police. So I had to suppress it, otherwise harm would come to me. Then I contemplated smuggling in the remedy I had given my landlady in the CM potency, so that it would cause her a severe aggravation. I felt in this case no one would be able to prove my involvement. But there was a split in my mind, because I felt I was misusing my medical knowledge.

[B/m/1,7/i]

- Tore up a greeting card a friend gave me, because I felt he is different behind my back. Then wondered if what I did was right or wrong.

[G/m/*,*/i]

- Felt sympathetic towards unclothed, helpless beggars. At the same time felt contaminated, and reacted violently if they tried to touch me.

[B/m/*,*/i]

- Was terribly frightened that some strange animal, side of me, would surface when I felt attracted to a bar dancer. Wanted the sexual indulgence, but was afraid that it would spoil the image I had of myself. Had the fear that I would lose my self-control and indulge in sex.

[B/m/1,2/i]

- Was unusually neglectful towards my studies. Then was irritated with myself about it, and about wasting time playing with friends.

[I/m/1,*/i]

- Unsure whether what I am doing is right or wrong, acceptable or not. Nervous feeling that others will think I am not a good person.

[G/m/1,∗/i]

Fight / Quarrel

▪ Felt tremendously attacked by beggars, and nearly started a street fight with them. Wasn't sure of my strength; made a very quick evaluation of it, as before a military exercise.

[B/m/3,∗/i]

▪ Feeling of being constantly attacked, so that I feel I can take out a gun and shoot without warning.

[B/m/3,∗/i]

▪ In a mood to fight, quite enjoyed fighting.

[B/m/2,∗/i]

▪ Was very, very angry at what I thought had been a breach of contract. At the same time was happy that I had a good reason to start an argument. Wanted to "finish off" the offenders with words and enjoy my superiority.

[B/m/2,∗/i]

▪ Felt like retaliating at any opportunity, at interference.

[C/f/3,∗/i]

▪ Challenging others.

[G/m/∗,∗/i]

▪ Talking of war.

[B/m/3,∗/i]

▪ Quarrelsome with family.

[I/m/1,∗/i]

▪ I felt that if I was in this state (of mind) any longer, I should take up a martial art or fighting skills to survive street fights, or take the first strike.

[B/m/3,∗/i]

Insulted / Looked down upon

▪ Felt insulted, patted off like an employee, when friends I had received from the airport asked me out for dinner.

[B/m/3,∗/i]

▪ Had the feeling that people were avoiding me because I was too thin. Felt that I did not come up to their expectations, that my behaviour was not acceptable. Felt inferior in comparison to others. Felt that others laughed at me. Praying that I should put on weight.

[H/f/1,∗/i]

▪ Feel insulted, looked down upon, treated as if I am nothing, of no importance. Was very angry, but didn't express it. Was disrespectful.

[J/f/3,∗/i]

Restlessness / Impatience

▪ Restless, wanted to keep on moving, to keep busy.

[C/f/1,∗/i]

▪ Restlessness indoors – could not stand. Wanted to go out.

[D/f/1,∗/i]

▪ Restless, impatient, wanted things quickly.

[D/f/3,∗/i]

▪ Impatient, wanted to finish things off, "cut-off" others.

[C/f/1,∗/i]

▪ Restless, unable to sit in one place.

[G/m/2,∗/i]

▪ Impatience – could not wait.

[H/f/1,∗/i]

▪ Impatience.

[B/m/3,∗/i]

Enjoyment / Relaxation

▪ Wanted to go out and enjoy myself.

[C/f/1,∗/i]

▪ Everything seemed routine, stupid and boring. Was easily irritated at this. Wanted to enjoy myself in the company of friends: talking, laughing, eating together with them. Was smiling, and a lot more lively.

[D/f/1,∗/i]

- Wanted to go home, relax and sleep.
  [D/f/2,*/i]

- Dullness, because no entertainment. Music ameliorates.
  [F/m/2,*/i]

- Want to roam, to enjoy.
  [H/f/2,*/i]

- Wanted to enjoy myself; was unconcerned about studies.
  [I/m/*,*/i]

- Felt this was no time to enjoy oneself, wasn't interested in attending any ceremonies.
  [G/m/*,*/i]

Miscellaneous
- Talking about the future.
  [K/f/*,*/i]

- Feel that I am being fooled, cheated. Feel that I should take revenge, do to others what they have done to me.
  [G/m/1,*/i]

- Revengeful.
  [H/f/*,*/i]

- Jealous.
  [H/f/*,*/i]

- Made it a point to bring a friend's mistake to his notice.
  [E/m/*,*/i]

- Fault finding. Feel others are wrong while I am right. Feel that others should listen to me.
  [G/m/1,*/i]

- Outspoken, sarcastic.
  [D/f/1,*/i]

- Possessive about my belongings, unwilling to share. Become sarcastic when asked to share.
  [G/m/1,*/i]

- Possessive, not sharing.
  [H/f/2,*/i]

- Felt taller than before.
  [E/f/*,*/i]

- Sympathized with a very high ranking "bad guy" in a movie. He had waited to get to the top, and then had taken his turn. I felt that I knew what it felt like to be a very high ranking gangster or mafiosi.
  [B/m/3,*/i]

- Don't want to mix with others.
  [H/f/2,*/i]

- Do things that I know are wrong despite realizing that they are harmful for me.
  [E/f/*,*/i]

- Felt like weeping on waking in the morning.
  [A/f/1,2/i]

- Sadness, on seeing one person shout at another.
  [E/f/*,*/i]

- Sadness from sister's problems (depression); wondered why this was happening only to me and my family. Feel as if she was slowly taking over the whole house.
  [F/m/2,*/i]

- Repentance.
  [G/m/*,*/i]

- More religiously inclined. Totally dependent on God with the feeling that he will do everything to help me.
  [G/m/1,*/i]

- Could take a decision without consulting others (very unusual for me).
  [A/f/1,*/i]

- More neat in working.
  [I/m/3,*/i]

Intellect

- Dullness of mind – was unable to think.

   [D/f/1,2/i]
- Absent-minded. Cannot recall what has recently happened.

   [F/m/2,*/i]

- Inability to concentrate on studies.

   [G/m/2,*/i]

DREAMS

Pursued / Behind

- I was being pursued by the mafia for not having paid a taxi driver who had tried to cheat me. The mafia had already "eradicated" two of my acquaintances, and I was sorry that I had not been able to warn them, and innocent people had had to pay for my mistakes. They were now after my family and me, with an intent to do us serious harm, to kill us. I had no concern about myself but wanted to protect my family members. The mafia was a huge crushing, overwhelming force to which I could not offer any resistance. There was no chance of getting back, no help. They had already broken into a family house where I had sought refuge. I had had to flee immediately from there along with my mother and little brother, because they could arrive any moment and take over. To escape them was impossible. It was a completely hopeless situation.

   I would have to cast off all previous connections, leave behind my name, and start afresh. For that, I would have to take the help of a powerful body like the State, but this was not possible, the mafia being too strong. Also, I felt that the State would not help me because it had been my mistake or crime. The only small hope was that some of my family who were away would escape.

I felt crushed by this overpowering force. I felt that such a tiny mistake could lead to such a complete catastrophe. It was frightful and horrible. I woke up chilly and freezing.

   [B/m/1,2/i]

- I was afraid of being arrested for the purchase of my new .375 revolver. I was unsure whether the gun was real or a toy because of its small size. But I was afraid to try it out because I might cause others harm. Then I realized that some gangsters had entered my house and they wanted to kill me. Felt at an advantage because I had a gun, but fled instead of facing them directly. They were pursuing me, and I hid in a big, dark garden outside the house by lying down on the grass.

   [B/m/2,1/i]

- I was being pursued by a man because I had committed a crime. I asked a woman for shelter. I ran first into her living room, but when he followed me there I hid in one bathroom and then in another, where he continued to pursue me. I felt a great fear of being caught, with palpitations, when he was close to catching me.

   [J/f/3,*/i]

- A man armed with a knife entered my house to harm my family members none of whom I could recognize. I had to protect them. He was attacking someone from behind. I managed to get the knife from him and bend it, but in the bargain got some cuts on my hands and legs, which were not painful.

[K/f/before dose]

High places / Falling

■ I was alone on a huge mountain, going higher and higher, when something flew just above my head. I tried to get behind it to catch it, but it disappeared. Then a hand came up from behind me and pushed me off. I was frightened.

[G/m/2,*/i]

■ I am a child climbing up a ladder that is very high in the air. The lower portion of the ladder is broken and can crack anytime. I am afraid that I might not survive. There is a rope nearby which I try to hold onto for security or support, although I know that it won't be of any help to me, should the ladder break. My situation is hopeless. I am scared of falling and feel I can't hold on much longer and have no strength in my feet. But somehow I manage to come down unharmed.

[B/m/2,1/i]

■ I had gone to a restaurant which tapered upward with each level. I was searching for place to sit. I finally found out that it would be available only at the top-most level. I had to climb a ladder which had no support with which to get up. My friends went first, and I was the last one to go. I reached the top-most step, and then slipped and fell. I felt that I had just reached where I had wanted to and then had fallen.

[E/f/1,6/i]

■ I was alone in a huge building which had many galleries. Outside there was a huge heap of stones as high as the second floor. I managed to find the door to the second floor after having encountered many closed doors, and jumped onto the heap. I was standing on top of the heap and looking at the sea around

me, when someone pushed me off from behind.

[E/f/1,7/i]

■ My grandmother was on a very high bridge. She fell off as she leaned to look over.

[H/f/2,*/i]

■ I was standing right on top of a tall, iron staircase that was hanging in the air, and that was without any pillars. I was afraid that if I took even one step to come down, I would lose my balance and fall down. I was paralysed with fear, was holding onto a railing. Was afraid also that my father and sister, who were standing on a parallel railing at that same height would fall. I advised them to be careful.

[K/f/1,*/i]

■ I was in Burma, where I kept climbing up a Pagoda [1] that was on a great height. Suddenly, we came down.

[H/f/2,*/i]

■ I was in a remote part of the mountains where I was being forced to stay against my will, but managed to escape.

[B/m/3,*/i]

■ A pregnant woman was suddenly thrown off the fourth floor. She died and I had been unable to help her. I wanted to stab the persons responsible as they were wicked.

[L'/f/*,*/0]

Fearful

■ My dead grandfather reappeared. I was happy to see him. Then he died again. My mother and I put him into a huge poly-thene bag, and took him to a far off place where no one would see us. When we opened the bag, all my relatives were present there. His face had swollen and his eyes were very large. Then suddenly he became very small and was foldable. I was very scared that this might be his ghost.

[H/f/2,*/i]

---

[1]   Eastern temple in the form of a many-storeyed tapering tower.

▪ A friend teaches me to ride a motorcycle. I am going at a very high speed when suddenly the brakes fail and the speed of the bike just keeps increasing. I am frightened. Suddenly a man with a cruel, frightful face appears in the way. I am afraid I will hit him, and am unable to avoid it although I try. He falls down, but when I look back I am surprised to find that he has disappeared.

[I/m/1,∗/i]

▪ Frightful dreams.

[E/f/1,1/i]

Alone / Left out / Neglected

▪ My friends, mother and sister were playing together while we were on holiday. They had left me out. They were walking fast, I was left behind, being slower. They had not included me in a single photograph, and I tore up all the photos. I was irritated even more when they were unaffected. I felt helpless.

[C/f/1,2/i]

▪ I was very angry at my sister and sister-in-law because they had decked up to go to a wedding without having included me. I felt that they were already married and since it was now my turn to be married, I should have been the first to deck up. I screamed, shouted, wept, was hysterical, but they did not react. I was trembling with anger, wanted to harm them but could not. I felt helpless and frustrated. I felt that they were being selfish and uncaring.

[C/f/2,∗/i]

▪ I was mad at my friends for leaving me alone during celebrations. I refused to join them when they later asked me to.

[C/f/3,∗/i]

▪ I was absolutely blank and shocked during an exam, because I could not recall any answers. I looked around at the others for help, for a push start. I finally gave up a blank paper. I got a score of zero in the same paper but scored of ninety-five percent in the other papers. The others were all staring at me, laughing at me, and seemed to be in their own worlds. I felt inferior, and felt that there was no one to care for me or understand me.

[G/m/2,∗/i]

▪ My relatives began to laugh because I was suffering from a fatal disease. I felt all alone.

[L'/f/∗,∗/0]

▪ A professor asked all the other students to go out and began to question me alone. I was very tense; he was asking me strange questions. After the lecture I went to meet a friend I was supposed to go out with. He had forgotten about our appointment and had invited other friends. I felt hurt and insulted. I felt angry but suppressed it, and felt neglected and uncared for.

[J/f/2,∗/i]

▪ My professor rejected an article I had written for a magazine, saying that it was not acceptable. Had the feeling that I was being rejected, not accepted.

[E/f/1,1/i]

▪ I realize that the train I have boarded is going in the direction opposite to my destination. I get off and board another train again going in the opposite direction. The train is very fast and is not stopping at any station. I am afraid that I am being taken very far away from my home, and that I will be late to reach home. I am also afraid that being all alone I won't be able to find my way home. A co-passenger consoles me and lends me money. Later, I see my father at a station where the train had stopped, with a sense of relief.

[A/f/1,1/i]

▪ I felt all alone and unwanted by my relatives who were ignoring me when I expressed a desire to join them for a trip.

[L'/f/∗,∗/0]

▪ My friends were not talking with me in spite of my requests. I felt betrayed, and felt that they do not accept me.

[H/f/1,*/i]

Helping

▪ I decided to fight for justice on behalf of patients who were suffering in a hospital from lack of proper facilities. A doctor there wouldn't allow me to. I told him to "get lost" because he was immoral and unfit to be a doctor. I asked the patients to support me, but strangely they did not react.

[L'/f/*,*/0]

▪ My alcoholic neighbour's previously large abdomen has reduced in size. He tells me that his abdomen has burst, and complains that his family will not take him to the doctor. I think he might have had ascites and feel very sorry for him. I get ready to take him to see a doctor immediately.

[A/f/1,1/i]

▪ My mother and I anxiously went out in search of my father who was very late in returning home. We met him on the way and he explained that he had been helping a very poor worker to sell off his land.

[A/F/1,1/i]

▪ People were killing each other with swords in a riot that had broken out. A small girl was being taken away, and her sister was pleading. I wanted to help her, but was unable to.

[L'/f/*,*/0]

Unfeeling

▪ I was alone in college and was reading the exam results that were displayed there. I had failed in all the subjects. It was unbelievable! I held my abdomen and began to laugh.

[D/f/3,*/i]

▪ I informed my friend that her sister had a brain tumour and only one month to live. I was not very much affected. My friend began to weep, but after a while resumed work without being too affected herself.

[D/f/1,1/i]

▪ I was to be operated for a heart problem. The doctor asked me to inform my family that I would require a pacemaker. My family laughed and joked about it when I told them.

[D/f/1,4/i]

▪ I see many lizards in my house without feeling very much afraid.

[E/f/*,*/i]

Danger

▪ We were far out in perfectly calm waters in a tiny, plastic dinghy. A huge wave, immense in the horizon was coming at us. I felt a huge fright. No one had predicted it. We would surely capsize and drown; there was no chance of getting back. But strangely, we managed to steer away and survive. Later, I handed the controls to a more experienced sailor. Then there was a strong current, but there was a ship big enough to take the storm in which we could dock. There was a huge danger that if we let go of the ship, we would drift away. I had to make the knot, but there was a danger that any second the motor below would be switched on, and I might get sucked in and die. I had to do it in a hurry.

[B/m/1,6/i]

▪ I was in a boat that was harboured on an island. Suddenly there was a very strong current that swept all the boats away from the harbour away into the open sea. Even with the most careful preparation and the best knowledge we could not have known about this current. We were left without food and without any water. There was no help. I felt hopeless, as if we would die. We were trying desperately to sail back to the harbour.

[B/m/1,6/i]

▪ I was furious at my parents when they accused me of being greedy for having eaten the last piece of a sweet dish in the presence of guests. I thought it was childish of them to have counted the pieces in the presence of guests. I felt that they were the ones who

44   Provings

were greedy, and that their anger was unjust-
ified.

        Later, while answering the door bell I
realized that my parents had installed an
elaborate double door security system. I
opened the door without much caution and
saw a huge German shepherd dog in the
darkness outside. Frightened, I slammed the
door shut in its face. I reopened it thinking
someone else might have been out in the
darkness. A man entered, and as I shut the
door I realized that my parents had shut the
second door to ensure their safety. I was
trapped alone with this man in the area
between the two doors which was of dark,
solid mahogany. I had the fear that he might
do me harm.

                                      [B/m/2,2/i]

▪ I was supposed to go alone to a particular place but I took three people along with
me. We were attacked by a snake while we
were there. My friend did not help us saying
that I was supposed to have come alone.

                                      [L'/f/∗,∗/0]

▪ Killed a person who I thought would
have killed me.

                                      [G/m/2,∗/i]

▪ I was joking with my friends and we
were joined by one of our professors. He
asked me to do something that was not proper,
or was unjust. At first I was unable to decide
whether to follow his thinking or mine. Later,
I decided not to follow him but was fearful
that he would harm me or emotionally black-
mail me if I went against him.

                                      [G/m/1,∗/i]

Sexuality

▪ Sexual encounter with a fourteen-year
old girl. Was feeling guilty because she was
innocent and a virgin. But she was making
advances, was very active and wild, and was
enjoying it. In the end, it was enjoyable, was
great fun.

                                      [B/m/1,6/i]

▪ Homosexual relationship with close
friend. I was disgusted when he asked me to
have anal intercourse with him, but did it
because he was a close friend.

                                      [B/m/3,∗/i]

▪ Called a fairly unknown neighbour
when I was alone and bored at home, to flirt
with him, and enjoyed it.

                                      [C/f/1,2/i]

▪ I was walking in a street when I saw a
few couples shamelessly kissing. I was embarrassed and shocked.

                                      [C/f/2,∗/i]

▪ My classmate makes sexual sugges-
tions to a professor who is wearing a burkha [1].
They have sex in front of us.

                                      [L'/f/∗,∗/0]

▪ Students and professors playing
Holi [2], and enjoying themselves.

                                      [E/f/1,7/I]

Threats

▪ I laugh along with the rest of the class
when my professor congratulates me for
having scored the least marks. Later I am
afraid that he will be biased because of my
scores and will fail me in my other exam. I
send my friends to request him not to do so,
but he does not listen to him. So I go myself
to request him, but again he does not listen.
I am angry because he is doing this purpose-
fully. I threaten him, shout at him, dare him to
fail me.

                                      [D/f/2,∗/i]

▪ Threatened, shouted at, and abused
a professor who had suddenly cut off my
friend's hair while they were writing an exam.
I ran to another professor and complained,

---

[1]   Loose garment meant to cover the body with
        a veil with eyeholes. Worn by Muslim women.
[2]   Indian festival when people throw coloured
        water on each other. Men take the opportunity
        to take liberties with women which are other-
        wise prohibited in Indian society.

but he wasn't affected. I again encountered the first professor, and he threatened to cut off my hair because I had abused him. I pushed him away and threatened that he "would pay".

[L'/f/*,*/0]

Miscellaneous

• A man was riding a bicycle which was quite similar to my stolen bike. But I could not question him, nor take any action for lack of any sound proof. I was surprised that he was riding it openly, not hiding.

[B/m/1,1/i]

• I was in a foreign country like Nepal where I was unable to rely even on products which had been manufactured in the West. I returned home to Germany where everything was reliable but had left behind all my belongings in Nepal. So I went back to Nepal, and had to pay a huge amount as airfare. I thought my organization was not good.

[B/m/3,*/i]

• I have searched many shops for a specific maroon T-shirt. When I finally find it and am about to pay for it, I realize that the sleeves are too long. I feel that just when I have got what I have been looking for, I lose it.

[E/f/1,7/i]

• Going into one shop after another until it is dark, and I realize I am late for my appointment.

[E/f/2,7/i]

• There was a lecture on gastroenterology being attended by very prominent, very important and highly knowledgeable doctors. Everyone there seemed prominent, important and "solid" – even the house physicians. I wanted to join in, to get the feel of the atmosphere of such an important talk. But I felt that they would not allow me because I was only an unimportant medical student, one among so many.

[B/m/1,3/i]

• A man asks me if he can join me on a sailing trip as a crew member. Later he takes charge of the whole boat. He is treating me like a fool. I feel he is controlling and imposing himself on me. I feel that all the fun is gone.

[B/m/1,4/i]

• I had to prove my nobility with my table manners to show that I was worth a relationship with a rich girl who lived in a fancy house.

[B/m/3,*/i]

• I had gone to the house of an old schoolfriend. He wasn't home and his housemaid was every suspicious of me. She was an elderly, noble, almost imperial woman. I felt she was trustworthy and reliable and had expected her to believe me when I said I was a friend of her master. I had expected a warm welcome, and wanted to leave immediately. But I thought that would make her more suspicious.

Then, a suspicious looking man entered the house and I wanted to protect her from him.

Another man who was a common acquaintance entered and she said if he recognized me she would believe me. But he pretended not to know me.

[B/m/1,3/i]

• I was at a wedding where the only person I knew was an old woman who has recently died. She had been noble, helpful and soft spoken in her lifetime. I was asking her if I could get her something more when someone called out to me. It was an old school friend who had been a show off and would always compete with me. I said if we had met earlier, we could have spent more time together.

[A/f/2,*/i]

• I walked out, being very much offended, when my parents mentioned an old girlfriend they had considered a bad influence, in the presence of an attractive woman.

[B/m/3,*/i]

- Was overjoyed to meet an old school friend, but she was hardly happy and reluctant to talk. She informed me that she was to be married the following week but was unable to invite me.

[A/f/1,2/i]

- A speeding bus is tossed up high in the air, and becomes topsy turvy. My younger friend says it looks very nice. Being older, I tell her not to say such things; someone we know might be in it. We realize the passengers are safe and that my father was amongst them.

[A/f/2,*/i]

- Was reluctant to stay in a village with my ailing grandfather, who is alone, and attend College there. Felt I would get bored.

[C/f/1,1/i]

- My father instructed me to wait for him in the car with my sister. I took the opportunity to drive. Was going zig-zag and avoiding people in the way, but felt it was easy. I thought I should stop, keeping in mind my father's instructions, but the brakes had failed. My sister and I managed to apply the brakes together and stop the car.

[A/f/2,*/i]

- Very excited at seeing snowfall for the first time outside my house. Ran outside, made a snowball and began to eat it, thinking it contained some minerals that were good for health.

A/f/2,*/i]

- I was in a house full of relatives. I found a room to change clothes in. My uncle who had been an alcoholic opened the door and entered. I was embarrassed and shouted at him, but he did not seem to take heed. Later my sister also entered, and people were coming in and out without paying attention to my words. I had to cover myself and look for another room. There was a lot of hustle-bustle in the house and no place to change.

[A/f/2,*/i]

- I was fearful of being wrong to answer a question that no one knew. The professor disregarded my answer with a gesture of the hand and listened to someone else instead. I was embarrassed and felt rejected. I did not look up at all after that.

[D/f/3,*/i]

- My recently married friend has given birth to girl twins. I feel that she doesn't have to bother about other pregnancies.

[A/f/3,*/i]

- Removed a surprisingly large among of dirt while cleaning the inside of my watch. It then began to work far, far better than before. Felt surprised, could not explain it.

[B/m/1,1/i]

- Was in a long queue outside in a bakery. A woman tried to jump the line. I did not allow her and managed to fight for my rights.

When I reached the counter, I asked for a cake which the shopkeeper broke into pieces using a fork before giving it to me. Was puzzled but did not protest.

[B/m/1,1/i]

- Was out to buy a book on snakes. Saw a book with the picture of a snake coiled up on its cover.

[B/m/1,3/i]

- Returned to the hospital where I was working after a four hour lunch break only to find that everyone else had finished their work and left. Felt guilty that I had not done my duty and hoped that no one had noticed my long absence. I decided to work the night to make up for the hours I had missed. But I needed a separate entry card to get through the security. I gave my mother's card and managed to get inside, but was afraid that if the fraud was noticed I would be treated like a burglar and be arrested. Once inside the hospital, I didn't seem to know my way around and got lost.

[B/m/1,6/i]

- I was in the U.S., high up in a skyscraper. The landscape below was beautiful; there was a lake with some sailing boats. But I was afraid to look down and wondered as to what would happen if I jumped off. I thought I should learn to parachute, but was scared at the thought and felt that aeroplane flying was a safer option.

Then I was invited on a sailing trip in rough waters. I agreed to go thinking it would be fun. But I felt ill equipped because I did not have another pair of trousers with me.

Later I had the urge to urinate and could not find a quiet place. I thought people will think it was improper to urinate in the open. Then I was unable to find my way back to the sailing boat.

[B/m/2,3/i]

- I convince my parents to buy me a very expensive pullover and skirt. Suddenly the skirt becomes very tiny.

[C/f/3,∗/i]

- Brushed my teeth so hard that two teeth fell off. They looked like glass pieces.

[K/f/1,∗/i]

- Eating a sticky substance so that my jaws are stuck together.

[I/m/∗,∗/i]

- I was trying to have terrible tasting tea which my mother had made. I couldn't tell her it was bad because she would be hurt.

Finally, I got up and told her it was bad and that I would make some myself.

[K/f/1,3/i]

- Recurrent, of being asked by professional dancers to join them in a performance, and later being appreciated by them.

[K/f/1,/i]

- Screaming at brother for giving up hope for his four-year old daughter who had a malignant brain tumour.

[C/f/3,∗/i]

- Suffering from hyperthyroidism; was very frightened. Woke up and checked my neck for enlargement.

[E/f/3,∗/i]

- Diagnosed as suffering from some disease during regular check-up.

[H/f/1,∗/i]

- Of events of the previous day.

[F/m/3,∗/i]

- Peace. (Before proving, dreams of war.)

[H/f/∗,∗/i]

- A woman and her husband are travelling in a train. The woman says the train will stop at the new platform while her husband says it will stop at the old one. The woman agrees although she knows that he is wrong.

[J/f/1,∗/i]

COINCIDENCES DURING THE PROVING

- Saw twins twice after having dreamt about twins.

[A/f/3,∗/i]

PHYSICAL SYMPTOMS

Generalities

- Increased thirst for cold water.
  [G/m/1,*/i]

- Desire for pungent food.
  [G/m/1,*/i]

- Aversion to sweets.
  [G/m/1,*/i]

- Pricking pain – right sided. Appears and disappears suddenly.
  [H/f/1,*/i]

- Draft of air aggravates.
  [A/f/2,*/i]

- Pricking pain left side.
  [H/f/2,*/i]

- Bodyache on exertion .
  [F/m/3,*/i]

- Weakness, as if I will faint.
  [B/m/3,*/i]

- Increased pulse.
  [J/f/*,*/i]

Particular symptoms

Vertigo

- Vertigo when riding: aggravated looking at moving objects; aggravated looking at stream of running water; accompanied by nausea.
  [B/m/2,*/i]

Head

- Heaviness in the vertex and forehead. Aggravated in the morning on waking; ameliorated after afternoon siesta.
  [A/f/1,2/i]

- Heaviness.
  [G/m/1,*/i]

- Hairfall in bunches.
  [H/f/1,*/i]

- One-sided pain, between 4.30 p.m. and midnight.
  [E/f/2,*/i]

- Constant headache, better clenching the teeth.
  [C/f/3,*/i]

- Heaviness in the vertex and forehead.
  [C/f/3,*/i]

- Heaviness in the afternoon.
  [L'/f/*,*/0]

- Pain in the evening.
  [L'/f/*,*/0]

- Pain in the evening.
  [J/f/*,*/i]

Eyes

- Sensation of heat.
  [H/f/1,*/i]

- Sudden, blank staring.
  [H/f/1,*/i]

- Drooping of eyelids.
  [F/m/2,*/i]

Vision

- Blurring of vision.
  [L'/f/*,*/0]

Ear

- Dull pain in the right ear, comes and goes suddenly.
  [C/f/2,*/i]

- Dull pain below left ear.
  [C/f/2,*/i]

Nose

- Sensation of heat.
  [H/f/1,*/i]
- Nose block.
  [A/f/2,*/i]
- Post nasal discharge: greenish, thick.
  [A/f/2,*/i]
- Icy coldness of the tip of the nose, from exposure to cold air.
  [E/f/2,*/i]
- Coryza, ameliorated in open air.
  [K/f/1,*/i]
- Tingling sensation with sneezing.
  [B/m/3,*/i]

Face

- Twitching on the right side of the lower lip, in the morning.
  [D/f/2,*/i]
- Rash.
  [B/m/1,*/i]

Mouth

- Bitter taste.
  [A/f/1,3/i]
- Sensation of heat.
  [H/f/1,*/i]
- White coating on tongue.
  [F/m/2,*/i]
- Increased salivation.
  [B/m/3,*/i]
- Dryness.
  [A/f/1,*/i]

Throat

- Pain, right side, at night.
  [D/f/2,*/i]
- Pain, left side, ameliorated from warm milk.
  [D/f/2,*/i]
- Severe throat pain. Worse: cold draft of air, swallowing.
  [C/f/3,*/i]

External throat

- Perspiration.
  [B/m/1,1/i]
- Itching.

Stomach

- Increased thirst.
  [H/f/1,*/i]
- Increased appetite.
  [H/f/1,*/i]
- Increased appetite but easy satiety.
  [G/m/2,*/i]
- Increased thirst.
  [L'/f/*,*/0]
- Nausea, on waking in the morning.
  [D/f/1,2/i]
- Nausea, with vertigo.
  [B/m/2,*/i]
- Pain in, and nausea with fever.
  [H/f/2,*/i]
- Nausea.
  [B/m/3,*/i]
- Nausea.
  [L'/f/*,*/0]

Rectum

- Crawling sensation in the anus.
  [B/m/1,3/i]
- Constipation.
  [C/f/1,*/i]
- Dark, blackish stool. Constipation. Worse eating bread and cheese.
  [F/m/2,*/i]
- Diarrhoea. Burning during stool.
  [B/m/3,*/i]

Urine

- Frequent urination, cloudy urine.
  [F/m/1,*/i]
- Frequent urination.
  [G/m/1,*/i]
- Polyuria.
  [L'/f/*,*/0]

Male genitalia
- Erection without excitement.
  [B/m/2,*/i]

Female genitalia
- Profuse, blood stained leucorrhoea.
  [C/f/1,1/i]

Respiration
- Desire to take a deep breath.
  [C/f/1,*/i]
- Suffocation in a closed room.
  [A/f/2,*/i]

Cough
- Continuous cough.
  [D/f/1,1/i]
- Cough, aggravated at night.
  [K/f/1,*/i]
- Cough, aggravated from lying down.
  [K/f/1,*/i]
- Cough, aggravated from talking.
  [K/f/1,*/i]

Expectoration
- Dark, blackish, in the morning.
  [F/m/2,*/i]
- Ropy.
  [F/m/3,*/i]

Chest
- Palpitations with nervous feeling.
  [G/m/1,*/i]
- Palpitations, could feel as if there was nothing in the body except the heart.
  [H/f/2,*/i]
- Palpitations.
  [L'/f/*,*/0]

Back
- Perspiration.
  [B/m/1,1/i]
- Pain in scapular region, and along the spine. Aggravated at night. Ameliorated in the morning. Ameliorated from hot bathing. Aggravated on exertion.
  [F/m/1,*/i]
- Pain, with inability to move.
  [K/f/1,*/i]

Extremities
- Pain, stiffness and a swollen sensation in the joints of the fingers, especially of the right hand, on waking in the mornings.
  [B/m/1,*/i]
- Numbness in right ankle; no power.
  [B/m/1,*/i]
- Pain in right arm, worse from lying on the left side.
  [F/m/1,*/i]
- Coldness of tips of fingers from exposure to cold air.
  [E/f/2,*/i]
- Cramp in the right foot.
  [B/m/3,*/i]
- Peeling off of the skin of the right foot and of the hand, in patches.
  [B/m/3,*/i]
- Pain in left shoulder, like a knife being stuck into it. Worse on deep breathing. Worse motion of shoulder and arms.
  [B/m/3,*/i]
- Stiffness and pain in both knees and the right elbow. Sore pain in thighs and elbows on walking.
  [D/f/3,*/i]

Sleep
- Sleepless between 4.30 a.m. to 5.30 a.m., but too lazy to get out of bed.
  [C/f/1,*/i]
- Intense compulsion to sleep in the evening.
  [E/f/1,1/i]
- Waking between 2.30 a.m and 3.00 a.m. to check if there was no theft.
  [F/m/1,*/i]

- Sleeplessness.

  [H/f/1,∗/i]

- Sleepiness throughout the day.

  [F/m/2,∗/i]

- Sleepiness in the evening.

  [H/f/1,∗/i]

Chill

- Chilliness, freezing after frightful dream.

  [B/m/1,2/i]

- Chilly, in the evening, before sleep.

  [E/f/1,1/i]

Fever

- Heat in the afternoon, between 3.00 p.m. and 4.00 p.m.

  [H/f/1,∗/i]

Perspiration

- On waking from sleep.

  [E/f/1,1/i]

RUBRICS

Mind

Single symptoms

— *Anger, eve-teasers, at.*

— *Anger, indecent behaviour of men, from.*

— Anger, violent, must restrain himself on account of fear.

— Cut, mutilate, slit, desire to, others, sharp knife, with a.

— Delusion, attacked.

— Delusion, attacked, people whom he had offended would gang up and attack him.

— Delusion, forced, that she is.

— Delusion, insulted, looked down upon.

— Delusion, talking, people talk about her.

— Destructive, alternating with fear of being harmed.

— Dream, alone, on a huge mountain.

— Dream, amorous, anal intercourse.

— Dreams, amorous, homosexuality.

— Dreams, animals, lizards.

— Dreams, animals, snakes, attacked by.

— Dreams, attacked, knife, with a.

— Dreams, body, body parts, jaws stuck together.

— Dreams, brakes failing.

— Dreams, catch, trying to, something that flew above his head.

— Dreams, caught, of being.

— Dreams, climbing a broken ladder.

— Dreams, danger, boat capsizing.

— Dreams, disease, hyperthyroidism, having.

— Drems, escaping from the mafia.

— *Dreams, falling, high places, pushed off, from behind.*

— *Dreams, falling, ladder, from.*

— Dreams, fighting for her rights.

— Dreams, friends, betrayed by.

— Dreams, friends, neglected by.

— Dreams, help others, unable to.

— Dreams, force, sudden, strong, over-whelming, and he could not fight back.

— Dreams, home, being taken far away from.

— Dreams, imposed upon, being.

— Dreams, improper, professor asking him to do something.

— Dreams, laughed at, being.

— Dreams, left out, being.

— Dreams, peace.

— Dreams, pursued, mafia, by the.

— Dreams, shameless.

— Dreams, snow, of eating.

— Dreams, threatening his professor.

— Dreams, twins.

— Dreams, unimportant, being.

— Dreams, unsuccessful efforts, harm others, to.

— Fear, animal, within him would surface.

— Fear, caught, of being.

— Fear, forsaken, of being.

— Fear, mistake making.

— Fear, punishment, divine.

— Fear, raped, of being.

— Kill, sudden impulse to, those who disturb him.

— Malicious, deceitfully.
— Sympathy, compassion, mafia leader, towards.

Common symptoms

— Absent-mindedness.
— *Abusive, insulting.*
— Ailments from anger, suppressed.
— Ailments from embarrassment.
— Amorous disposition.
— *Amusement, desire for.*
— Anger, contradiction from.
— Anger, laughing, followed by.
— Anger, trembling with.
— *Anger, violent.*
— *Antagonism, herself with.*
— Anxiety, conscience of.
— Anxiety, family, about his.
— Anxiety, future, about.
— Anxiety, health, about.
— Cares, others, about.
— Censorious, critical.
— *Company, desire for.*
— Company, desire for, alone, while, aggravates.
— Concentration, difficult.
— Conscientious about trifles.
— Contradiction, intolerant of.
— Cruelty.
— Cut, mutilate, slit, desire to, others.
— Dancing.
— Delusion, animals, snakes in and around her.
— Delusion, criminal, that he is.
— Delusion, deceived, is.
— Delusion, deserted, forsaken.
— Delusion, faces, sees, hideous.
— Delusion, great person, is.
— Delusion, neglected, duty, he has, his.

— Delusion, neglected, she is.
— Delusion, noise hears.
— Delusion, people, behind him, someone is.
— Delusion, persecuted, that he is.
— Delusion, sceptres, sees.
— Delusion, smaller, he is.
— Delusion, superiority, of.
— Delusion, tall, he is.
— Delusion, wrong, he has done.
— *Dreams, amorous.*
— Dreams, animals.
— Dreams, animals, dogs.
— Dreams, animals, snakes.
— Dreams, anxious.
— Dreams, astray going.
— Dreams, body, body parts, teeth breaking off.
— *Dreams, danger.*
— Dreams, dead people, of.
— Dreams, embarrassment.
— *Dreams, falling.*
— *Dreams, falling, high places, from.*
— Dreams, fights.
— Dreams, fleeing, of.
— Dreams, frightful.
— Dreams, killing.
— *Dreams, pursued, of being.*
— Dreams, riots.
— Dreams, snow.
— Dreams, war.
— Dreams, water, sailing.
— Dullness, sluggishness, difficulty of thinking and comprehending.
— Escape, attempts to.
— Fancies, lascivious.
— Fear, alone, of being.
— Fear, attacked, of being.

— Fear, danger, impending, of.
— Fear, death, of.
— Fear, evil, of.
— Fear, falling, of.
— Fear, ghosts, of.
— Fear, happen, something will.
— Fear, high places.
— Fear, injured, of being.
— Fear, robbers.
— Fear, self-control, losing.
— *Fight, wants to.*
— *Forsaken feeling.*
— Forsaken feeling, isolation, sensation of.
— Hatred and revenge.
— Helplessness, feeling of.
— Hide, desire to.
— *Hurry, haste.*
— Impulse, morbid.
— Impulse, morbid, violence, to do.
— Injustice, cannot support.
— Irresolution, indecision.
— **Irritability**.
— Irritability, trifles, at.
— Jealousy.
— Kill, desire to.
— Kill, desire to, knife, with a.
— Loquacity.

— Malicious, spiteful, vindictive.
— Mocking, sarcasm.
— Plans, revengeful.
— Rage, fury.
— Religious affections.
— Restlessness, nervousness.
— Restlessness, impatience.
— Rudeness.
— Self-control, wants to control himself.
— Shrieking, screaming.
— Shrieking, screaming, anger, during.
— Starting, noise, from.
— Striking.
— Suspiciousness, mistrustful.
— Suspiciousness, friends, to.
— Talk, talking, talks, war, of.
— Thoughts, persistent, evil, of.
— Thoughts, persistent, homicide, of.
— Thoughts, persistent, injury to others, of doing.
— Thoughts, two trains of thoughts.
— Threatening.
— Two wills.
— Unfeeling.
— Violence.
— Violence, deeds of, rage, leading to.
— Will, contradiction, of.

Physical symptoms

Generalities
– Air draft aggravates.
– Cold aggravates.
– Food and drink, bread aggravates.
– Food and drink, cheese aggravates.
– Food and drink, cold drink, cold water, desire.

– Food and drink, spices, desire.
– Food and drink, sweets, aversion.
– Pain, right side of body.
– Pain, left side of body.
– Pain, neuralgic.
– Pulse frequent.
– Restlessness.

- Swollen, sensation.
- Weakness.

Vertigo
- Looking, moving object, at.
- Motion.
- Nausea, with.
- Riding.
- Water, crossing, running.

Head
- Hair falling.
- *Heaviness*.
- Heaviness, morning, waking, on.
- Heaviness, afternoon.
- Heaviness, siesta ameliorates (single).
- Heaviness, forehead.
- Pain, morning.
- Pain, afternoon, midnight, until (single).
- Pain, evening.
- Pain, clenching teeth ameliorates.
- Pain, constant, continued.
- Pain, sides, one-side.
- Pain, pressing, vertex.
- Perspiration, forehead.
- Perspiration, temples.

Eye
- Heat, in.
- Heaviness, lids.
- Staring.

Vision
- Blurred.

Ear
- Pain, appears suddenly, and disappears suddenly (single).
- Pain, aching.
- Pain, aching, right.
- Pain, pain below the ear, left (single).

Nose
- Coldness, tip, of.
- Coryza, air open ameliorates.
- Discharge, posterior nares.
- Heat, in.
- Obstruction.
- Sneezing.
- Tingling inside.

Face
- Eruptions, rash.
- Twitching, lips, lower.

Mouth
- Discolouration, tongue, white.
- Dryness.
- Heat.
- Salivation.
- Taste, bitter.

Throat
- Pain, right.
- Pain, left.
- Pain, night.
- Pain, morning ameliorates (single).
- Pain, air draft.
- Pain, cold things, from.
- Pain, drinks, warm ameliorates.
- Pain, swallowing.

External throat
- Itching.
- Perspiration.

Stomach
- Appetite, easy satiety.
- Appetite increased.
- *Nausea*.
- Nausea, morning, waking, on.
- Pain.

- Pain, heat, during.
- Pain, nausea, during.
- Pain, pricking, left side.
- Thirst.

Rectum
- Constipation.
- Diarrhoea.
- Pain, burning, diarrhoea, during.

Stool
- Black.

Bladder
- Urination, frequent.

Urine
- Cloudy

Male
- Erections, sexual desire, without.

Female
- Leucorrhoea, bloody.
- Leucorrhoea, copious.

Respiration
- Sighing.

Cough
- Night.
- Constant.
- Lying aggravates.
- Talking aggravates.

Expectoration
- Morning.
- Blackish.
- Dark.
- Ropy.

Chest
- Palpitation, of heart.
- Palpitation, anxiety, with.
- Palpitation, tumultuous, violent, vehe-

ment, as if she had only a heart (single).

Back
- Pain.
- Pain, morning.
- Pain, night.
- Pain, exertion from.
- Pain, motion, on.
- Pain, warm bath ameliorates.
- Pain, dorsal region, scapulae.
- Pain, spine.

Extremities
- Coldness, fingers, tips, of.
- Cramps, foot, right.
- Eruptions, hand, desquamation.
- Numbness, ankle.
- Pain, upper limbs, right.
- Pain, upper limbs, lying on painless side (single).
- Pain, upper limbs.
- Pain, shoulder.
- Pain, shoulder, motion, on.
- Pain, shoulder, motion, arm, of.
- Pain, shoulder, respiration, during
- Pain, elbow.
- Pain, elbow right.
- Pain, fingers, right.
- Pain, fingers, morning, waking, on (single).
- Pain, fingers, joints.
- Pain, knee.
- Pain, cutting, shoulder.
- Pain, cutting, shoulder, left (single).
- Pain, sore, elbow.
- Pain, sore, elbow, walking, while (single)
- Pain, sore thigh.
- Pain, sore thighs, walking, while.
- Stiffness, elbow, right.

- Stiffness, fingers, morning.
- Stiffness, knee.

Sleep

- Sleepiness.
- Sleepiness, daytime.
- Sleepiness, evening.
- Sleeplessness.
- Sleepiness, midnight, after 4.30 a.m.
- Sleepiness, midnight, after, 5.30 a.m., until (single).

Chill

- Chilliness, evening.
- Chilliness, frightful dream after (single).

Fever

- Afternoon, 3.00 p.m.- 4.00 p.m.

Perspiration

- Sleep, waking, after.

THEMES

1. Feeling all alone, isolated.

    Feeling that no one understands her, that her friends don't care for her.

    Feeling neglected, unwanted, rejected by family and friends.

    Feeling left out, left behind, not included.

    Caring towards younger cousin, who she felt was alone.

    Desire to be alone.

2. Feeling insulted, offended.

    Feeling, looked down upon, laughed at.

    Feeling inferior.

    Feeling unimportant, as if he was treated like a fool.

    Feeling embarrassed.

3. Feeling attacked, and wanting to attack.

    Desire to fight.

    Fighting for his rights.

    Challenging.

    Talking.

4. Feeling that she was forced.

    Feeling that people were "after him".

    Feeling that he was being pursued by a huge, crushing, overwhelming force to which he could offer no resistance.

    Feeling that he had committed a crime.

    Feeling that a small mistake of his had led to a big catastrophe.

    Feeling guilty for not having done his duty.

5. Feeling that he was pushed off from a high place where he stood alone.

    Feeling that she had been pushed off when she had just reached where she had wanted to.

    Feeling a hand from behind pushed her off.

    Feeling she was pushed off, and no one came to help her.

6. Fear to be alone.

    Fear he will be attacked or harmed when he was alone.

    Fear ghost would harm him when he was "off-guard".

    Fear someone behind him.

    Fear gangsters.

    Fear of being killed.

    Fear arrest, police, of being caught.

    Fear divine punishment.

    Fear attack from behind to herself and her family.

    Fear attack from snakes.

    Fear of being raped.

    Frightful / cruel face.

    Fear that no one would come to his help when he was attacked.

    Fear falling / high places.

7. Danger, his boat capsizing from a huge, immense wave.

    Danger, being attacked and killed.

    Being unable to apply the brakes on her car.

    Fear of being blackmailed if he didn't do something improper.

    Threatening.

8. Anxiety about future.

    Anxious for loved one.

9. Possessive about friends.

    Mistrustful about friends.

    Old friend reluctant to talk to her.

Dependence on God, feeling that he would do everything, help him when he felt isolated, so that friends would realize his impoortance.

Did not need to consult others.

10. Easily irritable, wild.
Intolerance of contradiction.

11. Violent anger.
Sadistic pleasure from violent attack.
Wanting to "finish off".
Desire to kill, to stab, to cut, slit.
Violent anger at ever-teasers.

12. Two wills.
Revenge but fear of harm.
Ethical and unethical, right and wrong.
Sympathy alternating with violence.
Fear of losing self-control.

13. Feeling that everything is routine, and wanting to enjoy herself.

14. Sympathizing with high-ranking gangster.

15. Wanting to go home where he was safe.

16. Restlessness, impatience.
Wanting to "finish-off ", "cut-off ".

17. Revengeful.

18. Jealous.

19. Censorious.

20. Possessive

21. Sadness.

22. Unfeeling.

23. Noble / imperial.

24. Hiding
Escaping.

25. Searching for something, and losing it when he had just found it.

26. Teeth falling off.

27. Jaws sticking together.

28. Disease.
Large amount of dirt.

3

THE PROVING OF *DENDROASPIS POLYLEPSIS*
(BLACK MAMBA)

The proving of *Black mamba* was conducted in April 1994 with twenty provers. The provers were between the ages of twenty and thirty-five years. They were initially given a single dose of the drug and asked to note their symptoms. Prover G, M, N, O and R did not take the durg. Prover T had also recently participated in another proving. After noting their symptoms, the provers individually met with me once every week, for the next three weeks. Prover A and C required a repetition of the dose after the first week. At the end of four weeks, we met as a group, collectively discussed our symptoms, and finally I revealed the name of the substance to them. If they had any further symptoms they got in touch with me and I have made note of such symptoms and added them into this proving.

The drug was obtained from Dr. David Lilley of "The Lilley Pharmacy", Pretoria, South Africa. The biological name of the snake is Dendroaspis polylepsis. It was prepared from the fresh venom of a live snake, which was stirred into glycerine before being potentized.

MIND

Emotions

Alone / Forsaken

▪ Felt that her brother didn't care for her, and that her father loved her brother more than he did her. Stopped talking with them. Later when sick, felt she needed their help to recover; so resumed talking to them.

[K/f/1,∗/i]

▪ Felt I couldn't depend on others, no one would help me. Had to do everything by myself.

[F/m/3,∗/i]

▪ Felt one is alone, and has to do things alone.

[J/m/2,∗/i]

▪ Felt I could not rely on anyone, had to do everything on my own.

[S/f/3,∗/i]

▪ Felt looked down upon, alone, tortured. As if there was no one for me, I was left out.

[P/f/1,∗/∗]

Black depression

▪ Felt dull though my mind seemed active. It was a heavy state. Felt suddenly as if there was a black cloud surrounding me, overwhelming me. Feeling so sad – was thinking only of death and accidents, especially of relatives. Felt I must get out of this state, otherwise I will go down, and then I do not know what will happen. A feeling of being unable to fight this state.

[N'/m/1,2/0]

▪ Felt surrounded by a black cloud, by darkness. Anxiety and sadness. Great weakness; tired and sleepy all the time. No inclination to do physical work, to go out. Too much anxiety regarding future; felt hopeless, helpless, though all was clear. As if the power of decision had been taken away from me. There seemed no possibility of going forward. A feeling of great loneliness, as if no one really understood. No desire for communication, for relationships. Feel strained away from people, cut off. Felt life was a drag, not worth living (though no feeling of despair). Feel possessed by this overwhelming state.

[N'/m/2,∗/0]

▪ Very low moods, no desire to work, talk.

[F/m/3,∗/∗]

▪ Very depressed, weeping.

[K/f/∗,∗/i]

▪ Depression because I feel I can't cope: nothing can be done.

[C/f/∗,∗/∗]

▪ Low moods, depressed feeling.

[S/f/3,∗/i]

▪ Felt as if there was nothing left. Had no desire to live. Tremendous depression.

Weeping profusely from the smallest remark. Felt that others do not understand my hurt and my difficulties. As if my feelings were "crushed".

[P/f/1,∗/∗]

- "Black depression": As if I am going into a tunnel that is getting narrower and narrower, and blacker and blacker. I feel as if I am getting totally cut off from the world; no one really cares, no one understands, and it is no point in trying to make them understand. I wish I could go to sleep, and never wake up again. I feel that everyone only looks to his gain, and no one really cares for me; I am not good enough to be cared for. I feel others come only to get and not to give. I am faced with a very selfish world, especially towards me. I feel as if one by one all my close ones are getting cut off; they are selfish. I get a feeling of anger and hopelessness.

[O'/m/2,∗/0]

Unfeeling / Harsh / Insensitive

- Impulsively kicked my two-year old cousin very hard, insensitively.

[B/m/2,∗/i]

- Direct, blunt, rude to others. Aggressive, shouting. Didn't care if I hurt others, whereas usually I take the utmost care that I shouldn't.

[B/m/1,∗/i]

- Unfeeling. Quarrelled with my mother and said the worst things I could have ever said to her, although I knew she would be hurt. I told her that I felt troubled by her relatives and that I would trouble her so much that she would kill herself by the evening.

[B/m/1,∗/i]

- Unfeeling. Refused to visit a close cousin who had met with an accident saying that there was no need for it. Didn't care and went for a picnic the next day.

[B/m/3,∗/i]

- Didn't feel the need to pray for long life of my parents, as I always do whenever I see a dead body being carried away.

[B/m/1,4/i]

- Insensitive to people around me, to what they feel.

[A/f/ 2,∗/ii]

- Was unusually harsh to my grandmother, felt she is doing this to me since so many days.

[C/f/3,∗/ii]

- Was not touched by the news of the death of an uncle to whom I was very attached. I was blank, did not react. Felt it had happened just as it was to have happened.

[P/f/2,∗/i]

- Insensitive. Was angry about the train having been stopped, when a woman fell off while boarding. Did not feel any concern for her.

[Q/f/2,∗/i]

- Skipped my usual bedtime prayers without any feeling of restlessness.

[B/m/1,1/i]

- Use harsh, abusive language. No control over myself. Loquacious. Challenging others all the time; talking in a manner that would be hurtful to them without being affected myself. Not behaving in a civilized manner.

[B/m/1,4/i]

- Deliberately pushed a woman in the bus in such a way that she wouldn't know. Pushed her because I felt she was being egoistic.

[C/f/2,∗/ii]

Malicious

- Was irritable, rude, malicious and abusive with a servant because he had betrayed my father who had done so much for him. Felt he is low, I shouldn't talk to him. Deliberately did not give him any food and also tried to ensure that his brother did not get a job. Wanted to catch hold of him and ask him to get out.

[A/f/2,∗/ii]

- One female prover who had been disappointed in love developed a very vindictive attitude during the proving. Her friends reported that she had been making several blank telephone calls late in the night to disturb her former boyfriend who was now married. She also made several phone calls to the families of her former boyfriend and his wife, and posing to be someone else started to spread maligning statements about them. She was doing this deliberately and cold-bloodedly and seemed to derive immense pleasure out of it. When it was brought to my notice I questioned her about it, and she did not repent, had absolutely no remorse. This behaviour did not persist once the proving was over.

[Master prover]

- If someone irritated me, I retaliated, "gave back".

[P/f/2,∗/i]

- Angry if anyone overtakes me while driving. Widen my eyes, make an angry, frightening face and want to curse at them.

[F/m/2,∗/i]

Aggressiveness/Quarrelsomeness/Fighting

- Reacting in a rapid and aggressive manner. Was abusive when a friend said something about me which wasn't really bad. Would not listen to anyone; held my point of view obstinately even though there was no logic behind it. Answered rapidly and would not hear others. Excited during arguments, almost got out of my chair. Demanded that the other person look at me, listen to my arguements. Feel that others *have* to listen to me, to agree with me.

[B/m/1,3/i]

- A lot of aggression; I feel I can take on anyone.

[B/m/3,∗/i]

- Forced my point of view during a lecture. Snatched the mike out of the lecturer's hand and spoke loudly. Felt the lecturer was wasting time. Gave the example of a girl who was raped and compelled him to accept that it was her fault. My friends present thought I was aggressive, almost fighting with him, and were afraid I would have grabbed his throat had he contradicted me.

[B/m/3,∗/i]

- Attention remained constantly on a fight that I could hear from a distance.

[B/m/3,∗/i]

- Quarrelsome with family members. Though wrong, proved I was right and made them apologize.

[D/f/2,∗/i]

- Have been cursing at trifles. Cursed at a smoker and wanted to beat him up.

[H/m/2,∗/i]

- Irritated when someone is standing in front of me, as when travelling in a bus. Feel like beating up the person.

[S/f/2,∗/i]

- Am ready to take on anyone I come across: "Come on, let's fight, let's box." I feel I am behaving like an animal.

[B/m/1,∗/i]

Anger / Irritability

- Irritable on small matters – looked at brother threateningly because he made a mistake.

[F/m/2,∗/i]

- A lot of anger. Impulse to abuse and curse, but did not actually do it.

[I/m/2,∗/i]

- Anger that had been under control for the last three months surfaced again.

[J/m/1,∗/i]

- Though angry, unable to express it.

[P/f/1,∗/i]

- Anger, increasing and decreasing suddenly.

[R'/f/2,∗/0]

- Though angry internally, showed I

was happy on the surface.

[C/f/∗,∗/∗]

- Irritable and rude to strangers who would ask for directions.

[A/f/2,∗/ii]

Impulsiveness / Rash / Hurry

- Was impulsive in prescribing, without my usual feeling of restlessness about not having worked out the case.

[B/m/1,4/i]

- Impulsive.

[B/m/4,∗/i]

- Refused to listen to a colleague who was presenting a case. After two minutes of hearing him told him it wasn't taken properly and that we would talk only after he retook it.

[B/m/2,∗/i]

- Hurried. Would run instead of walk. Quickness of action as if short of time.

[P/f/1,∗/i]

- Have become irresponsible, and rash. Don't care about what anyone thinks of me, but feel bad about my behaviour.

[H/m/1,∗/i]

- Taking more risks than usual. Careless, reckless in driving.

[B/m/3,∗/i]

Harmed / Attacked / Tortured / Harrassed

- Felt tortured, harassed. I had had enough and didn't want anymore.

[F/m/∗,∗/i]

- Had the constant feeling as if someone was behind me. Felt he would come and touch me or harm me from behind. Yet never looked back – was unafraid – felt I would face him.

[F/m/2,∗/i]

- Felt those around me were trying to harm me, or were deliberately doing things to harrass me.

- While standing at the window, the idea came to me that someone would hit me

on the head with an object.

[H/m/1,∗/i]

- Was provoked quite easily when a powerful politician made a remark against a renowned scholar. Was wild. Wanted to find out his place of residence and kill him, irrespective of the consequences. I felt it was an attack.

[M'/m/2,∗/0]

Helping / Fighting for others

- Recollected some incidents I had forgotten about:

    – A drunken man had tried to force his way into a bus by which I was travelling. He had slapped a man who did not react. I felt the man could not take care of himself and I should help him. I had got up, pulled the drunkard out of the bus and thrashed him. He had later brought a sword and the police had to be called. I was only around seventeen years old at the time.

    – My friends had played a joke on a stranger. He asked me which one of them was responsible. When I had refused to tell him, he had started to beat me up. I felt it was wrong. I too hit back, and threatened him, "You hit me once again and I will beat you up. And if you come here again I will see that you never go back." Four people had tried to hold me back, but couldn't. I did not reveal the name of the friend responsible for the joke. I was stubborn. I felt I should take on a fight for my friends.

    – A man had thrown a stone at a small guy. No one else had said anything but I had gone forward and fought for him.

[B/m/1,5/i]

- Wanted to help a woman who was carrying a lot of weight.

[C/f/2,∗/ii]

- Weep when I see others suffering or even someone being helped.

[R'/f/3,∗/0]

Sexuality

- Was unusually cool while standing very close to a girl. Had lost my usual sense of self-consciousness and carefulness that I shouldn't touch her even by mistake.

  [B/m/1,4/i]

- In the evening, had an impulse to call out to an unknown girl and pass a comment. Have begun to feel an anxiety whenever I see a girl, as if I would pass a comment. Have to look the other way from fear of losing self-control. Felt that I am not behaving like a human being, rather like an animal. Felt a certain amount of guilt that what I am doing is not correct. Felt low and horrible about being unable to control myself, about my crude inhuman behaviour.

  [B,/m/1,*/i]

- Had the vision as if I had two penises. Felt surprised.

  [M'/m/3,*/0]

Courage

- A bit more courageous.

  [C/f/2,*/ii]

- Have become a bit more courageous.

  [D/f/1,*/ii]

- Took scoldings courageously, was stronger in tackling things. Held to my point of view.

  [P/f/2,*/i]

- Felt courageous. Had the impulse to climb out from the door of a moving train and get in through the window. Wanted to go trekking.

  [Q/f/2,*/i]

Snakes

- Vision of a coiled-up snake-like figure.

  [E/f/1,*/i]

- On closing my eyes, had the vision of a thick, brown coloured snake with black dots.

  [H/m/1,*/i]

- Have been talking a lot about snakes.

  [I/m/1,*/i]

Anxiety / Fear

- Felt the drug going through me into the extremities. Anxiety as to what would happen.

  [H/m/1,1/i]

- Woke up at 3.30 a.m., with a lot of anxiety about the future.

  [H/m/2,*/i]

- Depressed, wept a lot. Much anxiety about the health of parents. Felt mother would die.

  [P/f/1,*/i]

- Fear of high places.

  [A/f/2,*/ii]

Miscellaneous

- Am more patient while waiting, do not get anxious.

  [Q/f/1,*/i]

- Had the constant feeling as if something was going to happen. Felt as if there were too many people, a crowd, all crushing each other and I was trying to escape.

  [N'/m/1,*/0]

- Felt caged up, closed up, trapped, as if I had to carry out my work in that vicinity or area only. Couldn't go out of it. Felt jailed, restrained from doing things.

  [P/f/1,*/i]

- Feel I am doing wrong. Feel I am behaving like an animal, and feel horrible about myself.

  [B/m/3,*/i]

- While playing a joke on a friend, referred to him as my prey.

  [I/m/1,*/i]

- Have begun to believe that things should be either black or white – you can't stand in between.

  [B/m/1,4/i]

■ Had the constant feeling that I am not capable enough to do things.

[C/f/1,*/i]

■ Feel as if I am unable to cope up with my responsibilities.

■ Everything seemed monotonous.

[P/f/1,*/i]

■ Indolence, aversion to work.

[D/f/2,*/i]

■ Wept in the night, at bedtime.

[B/m/1,6/i]

■ Sentimental, sensitive.

[R'/f/3,*/0]

■ Ability to walk for long distance without any fatigue, or any realization of it.

[B/m/3,*/i]

■ Chattering, loquacious.

[B/m/*,*/i]

■ At 12.30 a.m, talked and made some gestures while still asleep.

[F/m/1,*/i]

■ Happy feeling, like a kick, like she is on a trip. Felt light, as if flying, as if on a high.

[E/f/1,*/i]

■ Very happy, at the height of my mood. Dancing.

[C/f/*,*/*]

■ Was fascinated with brightly coloured clothes.

[E/f/1,*/i]

■ While visiting a strange place, had the feeling that I had been there before, and had had this conversation before.

[F/m/*,*/i]

■ Was happy in the company of her father during high fever.

[K/f/1,*/i]

■ Desire to sit in my mother's lap.

[M'/m/1,*/0]

■ Awkward, dropping things.

[L/f/1,*/i]
[P/f/3,*/i]

■ Had the thought that I wouldn't attend a lecture on Homoeopathy, or even practice Homoeopathy which I am normally very enthusiastic about.

[B/m/1,*/i]

■ Was inclined to take the side of black people, especially in competitive sports. Sympathetic especially towards South African Blacks. Developed a hatred for white people.

[B/m/1,*/i]

■ Demanding in a loud voice that people understand me. Felt that people do not understand me, so I hurt them.

[B/m/3,*/i]

■ Felt like she was dying, with high fever. Wanted to make a will and bequeath all her gold and money to a close friend.

[K/f/1,*/i]

■ Contemptuous of others.

[B/m/1,4/i]

■ Was unusually critical of a teacher I found boring.

[C/f/1,3/i]

■ Told beautifully fabricated lies deliberately, for the fun of it.

[D/f/2,*/i]

■ Have become abusive, call almost everyone "dog".

[M'/m/2,O/*]

Intellect

- A feeling as if the mind was not working, a thought block. Aggravated from mental exertion, ameliorated from sleep.

  [B/m/1,4/i]

- Unable to recollect, or to comprehend what was spoken. Felt that I will never be able to comprehend. Felt blank. Knew the words but could not utter them.

  [C/f/1,2/i]

- Absent-minded, forgetful.

  [D/f/2,*/i]

- Absent-minded, took the wrong train (one that was going in the opposite direction). Absorbed in thoughts – got off at the wrong station.

  [Q/f/1,*/i]

- Absent-minded.

  [H/m/3,*/i]

- Much more thoughtful when taking a decision.

  [C/f/3,*/ii]

- Unable to concentrate on studies, despite repeated efforts. Kept postponing things repeatedly although I was convinced that they had to be done.

  [B/m/1,*/i]

- Numb feeling in the brain, couldn't understand what people were doing. Ameliorated at 4.00 p.m.

  [B/m/*,*/i]

DREAMS

Accused

- She.was wrongly accused of a murder that had occured when she was on a bus journey with her friends. She knew who the murderer was and had to stand up and prove that she had not committed the act.

  [K/f/1,*/i]

- I went to college one morning to find that everyone was accusing me of having raped a girl I didn't even know. They were all pointing fingers at me, accusing me. I felt a bit ashamed. The college principal began to question me. I insisted I was innocent, but felt that no one would believe me or take my part. I was alone, so I thought of a trick to get me out of this situation. I thought if a girl other than the alleged victim was asked to point out the person responsible, I might escape. Yet I was very frightened, so much

that I was afraid to go back to sleep after the dream.

  [M'/m/1,*/0]

- I was being wrongly accused of murder by a man who said he had some proof against me.

  [Q/f/1,*/i]

- A lady accused me of having bad intentions, when I was forced to hold on to her for support while jumping off a bus. My father tried to explain the situation to her. I felt guilty of being accused in the presence of my father.

  [F/m/2,*/i]

- I wasn't being allowed to enter college because some female students had complained to the watchman that I had been arguing the previous day. I felt I had been arguing for a good cause, and even if they complained they should have gone to a higher authority, and not to the watchman. I wanted a letter of apology from them.

[F/m/2,∗/i]

Deceit / Cheating

▪ A vendor wants to charge me a hundred and eighty rupees for a soda that costs only five rupees. I say I do not want it but he says that I have to buy it since he has opened it already. I feel very angry and am very firm. I feel that this is injustice and that this man is trying to exploit me, take advantage of me. He knows I am in need, and therefore I will pay.

[F/m/1,∗/i]

▪ My father was working with the secretary of our society to help him. I realized that the man was a smuggler and my father was being cheated. Our neighbour was looking at our beautifully furnished house, and commenting that it may be because of our connection with the smuggler.

[H/m/1,∗/i]

▪ I have picked up a pair of shoes in a departmental store. I start to put them on. One shoe is bigger than the other, and the sole of the smaller shoe begins to break. I take them to the counter. The shopkeeper says that he is unable to do anything. I feel cheated.

[H/m/1,∗/i]

▪ My friend tells me that his brother has been deceiving me by selling me perfume very costly. He advises me not to buy from him.

[D/f/2,∗/i]

▪ A bungalow owned by a very rich and important person is being robbed. The guards don't do anything although they see the thief. In fact they take some of the loot and let him go. The family inside the house shouts to catch the thief. The guards pretend to chase him but let him get away. They tell each other that they don't feel ashamed to do this since their master is a very rich man but gives them very little salary.

[H/m/2,∗/i]

Unfeeling

▪ Many domestic animals. My friend tells me that they should be tied so that they don't make a noise. We use a band to tie them. I get the thought of killing an animal and try to kill it. Then suddenly I realize what I am doing. There is no reaction on the part of the animal.

[A/f/2,∗/ii]

▪ I witness two accidents while journeying on a local train. One woman passenger fell off the train and died. Another woman was screaming to a man for help and she jumped off the train when he didn't listen. Also saw a corpse on the railway tracks. Wasn't really affected by any of these incidents.

[Q/f/1,∗/i]

▪ My friend was being murdered. I did not give a damn. Was escaping, being concerned only about myself.

[D/f/4,∗/∗]

▪ My teacher has a two-year old son, who is good looking and nice. He is not bothered about his child, is neglecting him. I feel sympathetic towards the child and play with him

[F/m/1,∗/i]

▪ Saw a ghost at the window. No feeling of fear.

[L/f/1,∗/i]

Fights / Battles

▪ I am involved in a gun battle in which a criminal shoots and kills all my relatives. I run out of ammunition and go into a house to get some more. An old person asks me how come I don't feel like weeping at the death of my relatives. I reply that I have no time to weep, though I feel it from inside. Just then I notice that my niece is sitting dangerously and is in the danger of falling. I hand her over to her mother and fetch the ammunition. I go outside and shoot the criminal. I know I must be careful otherwise I will be shot down by the police.

[H/m/1,*/i]

▪ War preparations – the main person was a doctor who was firm and right.

[C/f/3,*/ii]

▪ I had reserved a seat in a train, which my mother occupied. I fought with her.

[Q/f/1,*/i]

▪ My father says that he will divorce my mother. She says whatever he does is okay. But I fight with him. Feel what will become of us, who will look after us, finance us. Who would marry my sister and me?

[A/f/2,*/ii]

Irritated / Tortured

▪ An animal is kicking me, irritating me. Feel I should catch it by its neck.

[A/f/2,*/ii]

▪ I am being beaten up, punched. My lower lip is torn and bleeding. There is no one to help me. I am left out. Feel tortured, depressed. Feel I should retaliate.

[P/f/1,*/i]

Pursued / Behing him

▪ One of my friends had crossed the road, leaving the rest of us behind. Suddenly she was stabbed by a man who was totally dark. Then he ran after us to kill us.

[D/f/1,1/i]

▪ Was pursued by a murderer when on a journey with friends.

[K/f/1,*/i]

▪ I was searching for ancient coins in a remote place. By tradition no one was supposed to know about these coins. I asked some local vendors for help and they got out some coins from the water. Someone came from behind to stab me but I managed to escape.

[H/m/4,*/i]

▪ I was chasing some horse-riders up a bridge. When I reached the top of the bridge I realized that it was broken and the riders were below they all had fallen into the trap.

[M'/m/1,*/0]

▪ I was in a temple with my friends. There was a pond with crocodiles and snakes in it. I touched the head of one of the snakes just for the fun of it. It began to pursue me. I was really afraid, and woke up panting out of breath.

[M'/m/1,*/0]

Alone / Forsaken / Unwanted

▪ She was in a jungle where wild and tame animals were separated by a wired partition. The area with the animals was beautiful and quiet. A professor was guiding her group. She felt alone despite the presence of so many people.

[K/f/3,*/i]

▪ I have to attend the lecture of a professor I do not like. I force myself to sit in. I feel that the professor is not paying attention to me; I feel unwanted and I want to leave.

[H/m/1,*/i]

Helping / Caring

▪ Saw a person drowning in the sea. Jumped in to save him. Was bringing him ashore when a black trawler passed very close to me.

[B/m/2,*/i]

▪ I was alone with my sister who was in labour. There was no gynaecologist around for assistance. I had to conduct the delivery alone. The baby did not cry at birth and I became panicky.

[U/f/1,*/i]

▪ Our watchman comes to the door on Diwali[1]. Someone gives him food. I feel he has done a good work and deserves more.

[H/m/2,*/i]

---

[1]   Hindu festival of lights.

- I apologized to a fast friend for not having written to him in a long time. I enquired about his uncle who was my patient.

[J/m/3,*/i]

- I was weeping a lot over the death of my uncle. My brother-in-law advised I be taken elsewhere because I won't be able to take the shock.

[P/f/1,*/i]

- I saw a cute-looking child covered in a scarf. I thought she was dead. I called out to others to come and check if she was dead, but got no response. I then noticed that she wasn't dead, only debilitated. I picked her up, spoke nicely to her, made some lovable contact.

[C/f/1,2/i]

- My neighbour complained that his clothes get wet whenever I water my plants. I agree to shift my plants so as not to trouble him.

[M'/m/3,*/0]

Sexuality

- A boy I had known has returned from the U.S. He is wearing shorts and has long hair. He looks like a girl, although I know he is a boy. He is smoking and I enquire why he is doing so.

[A/f/1,2/ii]

- I was standing near a garbage dump when I saw a person surrounded by eunuchs. They were troubling him. One of them who was scantily dressed had put his arms around him (as in an embrace) and was holding him. Then this eunuch lifted the man up and began spinning /rolling him around. The man was trying to get out of his grip. He was asking for help. I was shouting angrily that they leave him, although I did not go to help.

[B/m/1,1/i]

- Two boys between nine and ten years of age were having a homosexual relationship. I was surprised because I felt they were very young.

[F/m/1,*/i]

- A famous model who usually appears in scanty clothing was "properly" dressed. She was playing hoop with a man.

[F/m/2,*/i]

- A man was massaging a woman's legs in a beauty parlour. I was horrified! Then I realized that the woman was me, my legs were transparent, and I could see my arteries and veins.

[G'/f/1,*/0]

- My friend takes me to a hill resort where many foreigners are lying around naked. I feel I cannot live in such a place because it is morally wrong, and also we could be sexually assaulted. My friend insists on staying there, so we split. But I call him back.

[H/m/2,*/i]

- A beautiful movie heroine tells the director that she wants to wear a low cut dress. The director says it is not required for the scene. The heroine feels someone should start the trend and she wants to do so.

[H/m/2,*/i]

- A movie hero was trying to physically assault her. She was taken to his harem.

[K/f/1,*/i]

- Am working in my vest and showing off my biceps.

[I/m/1,*/i]

- While travelling in the train, I realized that a monk had an erect penis. I was surprised but told myself that it was my mind which was like that, and blamed myself for being sexual-minded.

[J/m/1,*/i]

- Plesant dream of playing Holi[1].

[B/m/4,*/i]

---

[1] Indian festival of colours when people throw coloured water on each other. Men use this opportunity to take liberties with women, which are otherwise prohibited in Indian society.

Snakes / Animals

- A patient who has come to me for a consultation is wearing a white T-shirt with black and white squares on it (like a chess-board). I feel that I will think of a snake remedy that has the same theme and prescribe the same for him.

    [F/m/1,*/i]

- My father was telling me that *Vipera* should be proved.

    [I/m/1,*/i]

- I was bitten by a rattle snake while I was in the U.S. I started to feel benumbed everywhere except in the mind.

    [N'/m/1,*/0]

- Long, dark-green, spotted snake with a flat mouth, running very fast.

    [M'/m/1,*/0]

- I had participated in a competition where a wire had to be rolled spirally around the body, by making snaky movements. I made so many turns that people told me that I had won even before the competition was over.

    [C/f/2,*/ii]

- Her neighbour brought his pet lion into her house. She objected because it might eat up her pet dog. She quarrelled with family members because they wanted to keep it.

    [K/f/1,1/i]

- My pet dog was suffocating. I revived her by giving her something to inhale.

    [R'/f/3,*/0]

- My family members were trying to change the names of my two pet dogs.

    [R'/f/3,*/0]

- A dolphin is sliding up a building.

    [I/m/1,*/i]

- I am talking to a relative over the phone in such a way as to hide important facts from him. A huge Alsatian dog is harassing and irritating me. I have the feeling of wanting to beat it, but outwardly smile and say that it is not letting me talk over the phone.

    [H/m/2,*/i]

Disease

- Going from doctor to doctor because I was suffering from weakness.

    [D/F/1,1/i]

- Swelling of the right side of my face.

    [L/f/1,*/i]

- Talking to a person with tuberculosis.

    [R'/f/3,*/0]

- My father and brother had large blood-filled abscesses on their face and eyes, and were unable to see. I felt that they must have committed some sin, therefore they had them while I did not.

    [J/m/3,*/i]

- Of having involuntary diarrhoea.

    [R'/f/3,*/0]

High places

- My husband decides that my bunga-low be demolished and a skyscraper be made there. My clinic is now on the twenty-first floor, but I am still doing fine.

    [P/f/1,*/i]

- Falling off the edge of a mountain.

    [L/f/1,*/i]

Dancing

- Dancing with friends while we were on a journey. Enjoying ourselves, making mischief.

    [R'/f/3,*/0]

- Dancing with Michael Jackson; there were compartments made of glass. It was dark and there were many lights on.

    [R'/f/3,*/0]

- Successfully performing a dance.

    [T/f/3,*/i]

Importance / Influence

- A cricket match was being played on the roadside in which the better side lost.

I had a bald man's photo with me. I glanced at him and felt that he was unfit for the team but was in it because of politics and influence.

[H/m/1,∗/i]

▪ I was accompanied by a very powerful person into a very extravagant departmental store. The store people bow to him to welcome him and show him around. He acts like a king. They give him too much importance.

[H/m/2,∗/i]

Miscellaneous

▪ Car racing.

[B/m/1,4/i]

▪ Was trying to catch a train with my friend. We missed it. We ran from one station to another in an attempt to catch it, but missed it at every station. Seemeds to be running without any feeling of fatigue.

[M'/m/1,∗/0]

▪ Journey.

[L/f/1,∗/i]

▪ Everyone was celebrating Diwali but we were unprepared, though everyone else was. But I was sure that everything would be okay.

[G'/f/1,∗/i]

▪ Family, parties, enjoying.

[S/f/3,∗/i]

▪ Unable to choose from among the dresses a friend bought for me.

[D/f/2,∗/i]

▪ I am being beautified for an occasion while my patients are waiting for me. I am feeling I don't want to get this done.

[P/f/1,∗/i]

▪ Deciding what to wear to a wedding.
[R'/f/3,∗/0]

▪ My mother has fixed my marriage without my having seen the bride.

[J/m/3,∗/i]

▪ My friend tells me that I have to take his opinion on every case. I am surprised and feel helpless.

[H/m/2,∗/i]

▪ Success, accomplishment.

[T/f/3,∗/i]

▪ Talking on the telephone.

[D/f/1,1/i]

▪ Talking to myself.

[J/m/1,∗/i]

▪ Students presenting cases to their professor.

[L/f/1,∗/i]

▪ A huge wave comes towards me and falls on me when I am surfing.

[M'/m/1,∗/0]

▪ I was in Benaras[1] on a holiday. I offered milk to a small Shivling[2]. My husband who was accompanying me, offered milk to a larger one.

[P/f/1,∗/i]

▪ I am able to buy lots of things with a small amount of money.

[R'/f/3,∗/0]

▪ My sister-in-law comes to see me, but I do not talk to her.

[D/f/3,∗/i]

▪ Hunting for a rubric.

[T/f/3,∗/i]

▪ I am washing the face of a child on a religious occasion.

[R'/f/3,∗/0]

▪ I was in a slum. My maroon purse was stolen thrice, and all three times I recovered it from the garbage.

[R'/f/3,∗/0]

▪ While travelling in a train, saw that a man had died, and some of the passengers were trying to console those who had been

---

[1]   Ancient city in North India; a place of pilgrimage.

[2]   Phallic symbol of the Hindu God of Destruction, Shiva, who wears a snake around his neck. Hindus worship both the phallus and the snake as symbols of Shiva.

accompanying him. On the other side, good food was being prepared and served. I tell my uncle about the food, but he wants better food and goes in search of it.

[F/m/1,∗/i]

■ The hero and heroine from a movie are sitting together on a bench. The hero's father comes along and the hero makes fun of him. His father advises him to go on the right path.

[H/m/2,∗/i]

■ A lot of students tell a professor that they will not be attending his seminar because they are changing residence and cannot give their corrrect address in the enrollment form. Was surprised that so many people were changing residence at the same time.

[M'/m/1,∗/0]

COINCIDENCES DURING THE PROVING

■ Saw a mongoose on two occasions.

[F/m/1,∗/i]

PHYSICAL SYMPTOMS

Generalities

■ Felt weak, numb sensation.

[B/m/1,∗/i]

■ Weakness at the same hour everyday: 12.30 p.m. to 3.30 p.m. Ameliorated from sleep.

[B/m/1,∗/i]

■ Trembling.

[B/m/1,∗/i]

■ Absence of usual aggravation from fatty, oily food.

[C/f/1,∗/i]

■ Generalized cold sweat, worse in the afternoon.

[B/m/∗,∗/i]

■ Pains come on suddenly.

[B/m/∗,∗,i]

■ Bodyache worse in the morning. No strength. Faintness, almost unconscious with the fever.

[K/f/1,∗/i]

■ Increased strength; no fatigue. In-creased ability to walk long distances without fatigue.

[B/m/∗,∗/i]

■ Trigeminal neuralgia. Pains-shooting, forceful, throbbing, sharp.

[B/m/2,∗/i]

■ Weakness, terrible, on waking in the morning, at 2 a.m.

[D/f/1,2/i]

■ Pains, going from the right side to the left.

[I/m/∗,∗/i]

■ Feeling very weak – as if I am going to sink into the ground from weakness, and from the weight of my body. Weakness aggravated in the evenings. Would slide into a chair.

[I/m/∗,∗/i]

■ Desires spicy food.

[I/m/∗,∗/i]

- Desires very cold food, icecream; even ice-cream is not cold enough.

[I/m/i,*/i]

- Desires oranges, during fever.

[K/f/1,*/i]

- Desires cheese.

[H/m/2,*/i]

- Extreme weakness during menses.

[A/f/2,*/ii]

- Refreshed after very short sleep.

[P/f/1,*/i]

Particular symptoms

Head

- Sudden headache, one-sided in the initial part of sleep. Was about to scream with pain when it disappeared.

[F/m/1,*/i]

- Severe pain right temporal region at 11.30 p.m. Sharp pain aggravated from talking; slightly ameliorated from keeping quiet.

[B/m/1,*/i]

- Pain, throbbing, with eye pain. Of sudden onset.

[D/f/*,*/i]

- Pain, burning, in the forehead aggravated at 5 p.m.

[K/f/1,*/i]

- Sensation as if head would burst with fever.

[K/f/1,*/i]

- Severe left-sided pain from loss of sleep.

[L/f/1,*/i]

- Pain – dull/sharp aggravated from talking. At 12.25 p.m., a vague sensation in the head, as if it was rolling, as if it had become very light. Felt numb, as if there was no sensation in the head. Ameliorated at 4 p.m.

Weak, numb sensation as if head would fall down any moment; had to support forehead with hand. Unable to concentrate with the pain.

[B/m/1,*/i]

- Dull headache throughout the week.

[U/f/1,*/i]

- Heaviness in right temple.

[R'/f/*,*/0]

Vertigo

- Giddiness and fear of high places.

[A/f/2,*/ii]

Eye / Vision

- Drooping of eyelids as if about to close.

[B/m/1,*/i]

- Photophobia.

[L/f/1,*/i]

- Eyes burning during fever.

[K/f/1,*/i]

- Saw figures on closing eyes.

Nose

- Sneezing, worse at 4 p.m.

[I/m/1,*/i]

- Coryza – greenish, yellow mucus, cold progressed very fast.

[I/m/1,*/i]

- Boil in left nostril – painful when inhaling.

[A/f/2,*/ii]

- Running coryza, nose block. Irritation in the nose.

[B/m/*,*/i]

Face

- Heat of the face.

[I/m/*,*/i]

- Pain at angle of jaw; sharp pain in right

cheek, at 3.00 p.m. Trigeminal neuralgia.

[B/m/2,*/i]

Mouth

- Pain in the right side of soft palate, aggravated at 4.00 p.m.

[I/m/1,*/i]

- Tongue: protuding out frequently.

[M'/m/*,*/0]

Teeth

- Sensitiveness of lower incisors – left side. Aggravated in the evening, until night. Aggravated from cold water. Aggravated from inhaling cold air.

[F/m/1,*/i]

Throat, external throat

- Neck pain. Worse in the morning. Ameliorated from rotating the head in a circular manner.

[B/m/2,*/i]

- Sharp pain in the right side of neck.

[B/m/*,*/i]

- Pain in the right side of the throat extending to the right ear, after eating fried food. Aggravated from empty swallowing. Aggravated while eating. Aggravated while drinking. Ameliorated on blocking the right ear with finger. Ameliorated drinking hot tea with brandy.

Had difficulty in opening my mouth due to the throat pain.

[R'/f/*,*/0]

- Pain, shooting, extending to the right temple.

[R'/f/*,*/0]

- Stiffness of neck next day after taking dose – movements of the neck were difficult.

[J/m/1,1/i]

Stomach

- Copious vomitting at night, with high fever.

[K/f/1,*/i]

Abdomen

- Pulsations in the epigastrium.

[B/m/1,*/i]

- Flatulence.

[L/f/*,*/i]

- Pain in lower abdomen before urination, ameliorated after urination.

[C/f/1,1/i]

Stool

- Diarrhoea, watery, with much flatulence. Aggravated in the morning.

[J/m/*,*/i]

Male

- Sexual desire increased. Intense desire to masturbate.

[M'/m/*,*/0]

Female

- Menses: early; scanty.

[C/f/1,*/i]

- Menses ten days earlier, associated with extreme weakness on the first day.

[A/f/2,*/ii]

Larynx / Trachea

- Hoarseness of voice at 1.00 p.m.

[A/f/1,*/i]

- Sore throat.

[G'/f/*,*/0]

Cough

- Hacking cough beginning at 1.00 p.m., disappearing by evening time.

[A/f/1,*/i]

- Cough after having taken only one sip of a cold drink.

[B/m/*,*/i]

Chest

- Palpitations aggravated in the afternoon.

[B/m/1,*/i]

- Chest pain, dull, worse right side, at

3.15 p.m., continuously for fifteen to twenty minutes.

[B/m/2,*/i]

Back / Neck

- At night, developed a pain in the left side of the back which was continuous, and came only when lying down.

[B/m/*,*/i]

Extremities

- Weakness in limbs.

[B/m/1,*/i]

- Trembling of legs.

[B/m/1,1/i]

- Cold sweat over shin, worse in the afternoon.

[B/m/1,1/i]

- Sensation of weakness, as if the bone was hanging vertically from the joints, while sleeping.

[I/m/*,*/i]

- Awkward, dropping things.

[L/f/*,*/i]

- About three hours after taking the first dose, pain in left shoulder (deltoid region), continuously. Ameliorated by some motion of the arm. Would come up again if the arm was kept in that same position.

[B/m/1,1/i]

- Pain in right toe, thighs.

[B/m/*,*/i]

Sleep

- Sleeplessness before menses. (Usually feel sleepy.)

[C/f/1,*/i]

- Before the proving, had been sleepless most nights. After the first dose, slept well for at least three nights, and especially on the first day.

[A/f/1,*/i]

- Woke up from sleep at 12.30 a.m., talked to someone, made some gestures, then returned to sleep.

[F/m/*,*/i]

- Sleepiness with weakness. While sleeping, felt as is bones were hanging vertically from joints.

[I/m/*,*/i]

- Sleepiness.

[R'/f/*,*/0]

- Sleepiness.

[M'/m/*,*/0]

- Feeling sleepy and weak.

[S/f/*,*/i]

- Excessive sleepiness – even if I get two minutes, would like to go to sleep.

[I/m/*,*/i]

- Sleepless, tossing and turning in bed. Could sleep only for two hours. Waking fresh after two hours of sleep.

[P/f/1,*/i]

Chill / Fever / Perspiration

- Fever 103 degree F. Bed felt hot, tried to search for a cool place.

[K/f/1,*/i]

- Typhoid fever.

[K/f/1,*/i]

RUBRICS

Mind

Single symptoms

— Abusive, insulting, calls everyone a dog.
— Anger, trembling, with legs, of.
— Clothes, desires to wear, striking, bright, vivid.
— Company, desire for, fever, during.
— Deceitfulness, avoids blame.
— *Delusion, black cloud surrounds him.*
— Delusion, caged.
— Delusion, inhuman, animal-like.
— Delusion, isolated, cut-off from others.
— Delusion, penises, he had two.
— Delusion, take on anyone he can.
— Delusion, trapped.
— Delusion, understood, she was not being.
— Dreams, accidents, being unaffected by.
— Dreams, alone, of feeling.
— Dreams, animals, kicking her.
— Dreams, animals, crocodiles.
— Dreams, animals, dog, harassed by.
— Dreams, animals, dolphins.
— Dreams, animals, lions.
— Dreams, animals, snakes, black and white.
— Dreams, animals, snakes, pursued by.
— Dreams, body, body parts, face, abscesses covered with, large, bloody.
— Dreams, body, body parts, face, swollen, right.
— Dreams, boy who looks like a girl.
— Dreams, car racing.
— Dreams, cheated, of being.
— Dreams, children, caring for debilitated child.
— Dreams, children, neglecting child.
— Dreams, childbirth, she had to conduct a delivery alone.
— Dreams, consoling relatives of dead person.
— Dreams, cooperating with complaining neighbour.
— Dreams, danger, stabbed from behind, of being.
— Dreams, deceitful, of being.
— Dreams, defending relatives.
— Dreams, doctors, consulting many, in succession.
— Dreams, drowning, saving a drowning man.
— Dreams, escaping, unconcerned about friend who was being murdered.
— Dreams, eunuchs.
— Dreams, exploited, of being.
— Dreams, father, advising son to take correct path.
— Dreams, homosexuality, amongst children.
— Dreams, killing, animals.
— Dreams, man, massaging woman's legs.
— Dreams, model.
— Dreams, monk, with erection.
— Dreams, murdered, he was to be.
— Dreams, people, powerful, important.
— Dreams, people, scantily dressed.
— Dreams, pursued being, murderers, by.

— Dreams, pursuing, of.

— Dreams, quarrels, mother, with.

— Dreams, robbery, guards, assisting a.

— Dreams, running without fatigue.

— Dreams, searching for ancient, secret treasure.

— Dreams, suffocation, reviving suffocating dog.

— Dreams, tortured, of being.

— Dreams, trap.

— Dreams, water, wave, huge approaching.

— Estranged, cut-off, feels.

— Exertion physical, ability for, increased.

— Fight wants to, defenseless, helpless people, for.

— Fight wants to, boxing, desire for.

— Guilt, animal or inhuman behaviour, about.

— Impulsive, alternating with fear of losing control.

— Impulse, climb out of running train, to.

— Impulse, hurt others, to.

— Impulse, tease women sexually, to.

— Quarrelsomeness, family, with.

— Reproaches, himself, sexual thoughts about.

— Sadness, melancholy, overwhelming.

— Sadness, melancholy, thoughts, death, of.

— Sympathy, compassion, black persons, for.

— Speed, desire for.

— Thoughts, accidents, of.

Common symptoms

— Abrupt.

— Absent-mindedness.

— Absorbed, buried in thought.

— Abusive, insulting

— Ailments, from anger, suppressed.

— *Anger, irascibility*.

— Anger, contradiction, from.

— Anger, sudden.

— Anger, violent.

— Answers, abruptly, curtly, shortly.

— Answers, hastily.

— Answers, violently, as if angry.

— Antagonism, herself, with.

— Anxiety, family about his.

— Anxiety, future, about.

— Awkwardness.

— Censorious, critical.

— Cheerfulness, simulates hilarity while he feels wretched.

— Concentration, difficult.

— Confidence, want of self.

— Confusion of mind.

— Contradict, disposition to.

— Contradiction, intolerant of.

— Courageous.

— Cruelty, brutality, inhumanity.

— Cursing, swearing.

— Dancing.

— Death, presentiment of.

— Death, thoughts of.

— Deceitful, sly.

— *Delusion, alone always*.

— Delusion, animals, of, snakes in and around her.

— Delusion, death approaching.

— *Delusion, deserted, forsaken*.

— Delusion, experienced, before, thought, everything had been.

— Delusion, flying, he or she is.

— Delusion, injury, about to receive.

— Delusion, light, incorporeal, imma-

terial, he is.
— Delusion, people, behind him, some-one is.
— Delusion, persecuted, that he is.
— Delusion, strong, he is.
— Delusion, tormented, he is.
— Dictatorial, domineering, dogmatical, despotic.
— Dreams, accidents.
— Dreams, accusations, crime, wrongful, of.
— *Dreams, animals.*
— Dreams, animals, dogs.
— Dreams, animals, killing.
— Dreams, animals, snakes.
— Dreams, animals, snakes, biting him.
— Dreams, battles.
— Dreams, beaten, being.
— Dreams, dancing.
— Dreams, death, of.
— Dreams, drowning, drowning, man, of a.
— Dreams, falling, height, from a.
— Dreams, food.
— Dreams, frightful.
— Dreams, ghosts.
— Dreams, journeys.
— Dreams, movie stars (*Coca-Cola, Lac leoninum*).
— Dreams, murder.
— Dreams, nakedness.
— Dreams, parties.
— Dreams, rape, threats of rape.
— Dreams, robbers.
— Dreams, robbing.
— Dreams, wars.
— Dreams, water, waves, of high.
— Dreams, weeping.

— Dullness, sluggishness, difficulty of thinking and comprehending.
— Dullness, sluggishness, afternoon, 4 p.m. ameliorates.
— Dullness, sluggishness, sleep, after.
— Escape, attempts to.
— Excitement, excitable.
— Exertion, mental, aggravates.
— Extremes, goes to.
— Fear, happen, something will.
— Fear, high places.
— Fear, insanity, of losing his reason.
— *Fight, wants to.*
— Forsaken feeling.
— Harshness, rough.
— Hurry, haste.
— Hurry, haste, walking, while.
— *Impulse, violence, to do.*
— Impulsive.
— Indifference, loved ones, to.
— Indolence, aversion to work.
— *Irritability.*
— Irritability, trifles, at.
— Kicks.
— Kill, desire to.
— Kill, desire to, person that contradicts her.
— Kill, sudden impulse to.
— Liar.
— Loathing, life, of.
— Loquacity.
— Malicious, spiteful, vindictive.
— Memory, weakness, loss, of.
— Obstinate.
— Procrastinating.
— Quarrelsomeness, scolding.
— Rashness.
— Rudeness.

— Sadness, melancholy, depression of mind, dejection.
— Sensitive, oversensitive.
— Sentimental.
— Shrieking, screaming, shouting.
— Suspiciousness.
— Sympathetic, compassionate.

— Talk, indisposed to, desire to be silent, taciturn.
— Thoughts, thoughtful.
— Threatening.
— Unfeeling.
— Weeping, tearful mood.
— Weeping, tearful mood, night.

Physical symptoms

Generalities

– Faintness, fever, during.
– Food and drink, cheese, desire.
– Food and drink, cold food, desire.
– Food and drink, ice-cream desire.
– Food and drink, oranges, desire.
– Food and drink, spices, desire.
– Pains, appear suddenly.
– Pains, neuralgic.
– Pains, shooting.
– Pulsation, internally.
– Sides, right, then left side.
– Sleep, short sleep ameliorates.
– Strength, sensation of.
– Trembling, externally.
– Warmth aggravates.
– Weakness.
– Weakness, noon, 12.30 a.m. to 3.30 p.m. until (single).
– Weakness, midnight, after, 2 a.m.
– Weakness, evening.
– Weakness, evening, sliding into bed (single).

Vertigo

– Vertigo, noon.
– Vertigo, high places.

Head

– Heaviness, temples, right (single).
– Numbness, sensation of.
– Pain.
– Pain, sleep, during.
– Pain, sides, left.
– Pain, sides, sleep, loss of (single).
– Pain, temples, right.
– Pain, temples, forenoon.
– Pain, temples, talking.
– Pain, burning, forehead.
– Pain, burning, afternoon, 5 p.m. (single).
– Pain, bursting.
– Pain, bursting, fever, with.
– Pain, dull.
– Pain, dull, talking aggravates (single).
– Pain, sharp.
– Pulsating.
– Pulsating, accompanied by eye-pain (single).
– Pulsating, sudden (single).
– Weakness, noon.

Eyes

– Closing the eyes, desire to.
– Pain, burning.
– Photophobia.

Nose
- Coryza.
- Discharge, yellowish-green.
- Obstruction.
- Sneezing, afternoon, 4 p.m. (single).

Face
- Eruptions, nose, inside, left.
- Heat.
- Pain, cheek, right, afternoon, 3 p.m. (single).
- Pain, jaw, articulation.
- Pain, neuralgic.

Mouth
- Pain, palate, afternoon, 4 p.m. (single).
- Protruding, tongue.

Teeth
- Sensitive, evening.
- Sensitive, cold, to.
- Sensitive, cold water, to.
- Sensitive, incisors.

Throat
- Pain, right.
- Pain, drinking aggravates.
- Pain, drinks, warm, ameliorate.
- Pain, eating, while.
- Pain, stopping ear with finger ameliorates (single).
- Pain, swallowing, empty, on.
- Pain, extending to ear.
- Pain, stitching, extending to temple (single).

External throat
- Pain, sharp, side, right.

Stomach
- Vomiting, heat, during.
- Pulsation.

Abdomen
- Flatulence.
- Pain, urination, before.
- Pain, urination ameliorates.
- Pain, hypogastrium.

Rectum
- Diarrhoea, morning

Stool
- Watery.

Male genitalia / Sex
- Masturbation, disposition to.
- Sexual desire, increased.

Female genitalia / Sex
- Menses, frequent.
- Menses, scanty.

Larynx and trachea
- Pain, sore.
- Voice, hoarseness.

Cough
- Noon, evening, until.
- Cold drinks.
- Hacking.

Chest
- Pain.
- Pain, afternoon, 3 p.m.
- Pain, sides, right.

Back
- Pain, left.
- Pain, night.
- Pain, lying, while.
- Pain, cervical region.
- Pain, cervical, morning.
- Pain, cervical, motion, ameliorates, circular (single).
- Stiffness, cervical region.

Extremities

- Awkwardness, hands, drops things.
- Pain, shoulder, left.
- Pain, thighs.
- Pain, toes, first, right.
- Perspiration, leg, tibia, over (single).
- Perspiration, leg, cold.
- Trembling, legs.
- Weakness.
- Weakness, sleep, during, as if bones hang vertically from the joints (single).

Sleep

- Disturbed, midnight (single).
- Restless.
- Sleepiness.
- Sleeplessness.
- Sleeplessness, menses, before.

Perspiration

- Afternoon.
- Cold.

THEMES

1. **Sexuality**
   A boy who looks like a girl.
   Eunuchs (confusion of sex).
   Homosexuality.
   The covert sexuality of seemingly saint-
   ly people.
   Nakedness, exposing oneself.
   Scanty clothes.
   Eve teasing.
   Sexuality among children.
   Feeling as if he had two penises.

2. **Agressiveness**
   Retaliation.
   Abusive.
   Cursing.
   Striking.
   Desire to fight.
   Arguing.
   Harsh.
   Boxing.
   Anger with trembling of legs and cold
   sweat.
   Malicious.
   Fighting with family members.
   Calling people "dog"
   Provoked easily.

3. **Wrongly accused**
   Blamed for murder.
   Accused of rape.
   Feels he has to prove he has not done a
   crime.
   Accused of sexual assault.

4. **Unfeeling / Cold-blooded / Hard-hearted**
   Not affected by death or accidents.
   Not caring about sentiments of close
   relatives.
   Feels as if he doesn't need God.

5. **Alone / Forsaken**
   There is no one for me.
   Courageous and independent.
   Left out no one to help me: have to try
   to get a solution on my own.
   Jailed.
   Caged.
   Great lonliness as if really no one under-
   stands.
   No desire for communication.

6. Fashion show.
   Bright coloured dresses
   Vivid design.
   Dancing – on stage.
   Beauty contest.
   Michael Jackson.
   Beautifully decorated house.

7. As if someone behind me.
   Feeling somebody will hit his head with
   an object.
   A watchman cheating his own master.

8. Tortured feeling.
   Feels harassed, people are trying to
   harm me.

9. Black / White.

10. Déjà-vu phenomena.

11. **Snakes / Animals**
    Dreams of snake pursuing him.
    Dreams of black and white snakes.
    Dreams of crocodile.
    Dreams of long spotted dark green
    snake being bitten by rattle snake.
    Dreams of animals.
    Dreams of killing animals.
    Dreams of killing animals by catching
    its neck.

12. Car racing.
    Impulse to walk long distances without tiredness.
    Fresh after two hours of sleep.
    Reckless driving.

13. **Black depression**
    Feeling of a black cloud surrounding him.
    Feeling he can't get out of it. Overwhelming anxiety about future, hopeless, helpless.
    Extreme physical weakness.
    Life is a drag; it's worthless to live.
    A very strong state has possessed me.

14. **Helping / Saving others**
    To help friend from drowning.
    To help relative in labour.
    Fighting for one's relatives.

15. Absent-minded.

16. **Deceitful**
    Lying
    Pretending to be happy when inside she is sad.
    Warns others but avoids being blamed.

17. Feeling horrible about oneself.
    Impulsiveness and fear of loosing control.
    Wanting to do something but not doing it.
    Blaming oneself for sexual thoughts.
    Considering oneself inhuman; feeling like an animal.

4

A PROVING OF *LAC CAPRINUM* (GOAT'S MILK)

In March 1994, a proving of goat's milk was conducted with four provers other than myself. None of them knew what was being proved. They were between the ages of twenty and thirty-five years. They were given four doses of the 30 C potency, with instructions to take them until the onset of symptoms or dreams. Prover E did not take the dose.

The drug was obtained from "VSM Pharmacy", Holland. It had been prepared by Dr. Kees Dam, Amsterdam.

MIND

Emotions

Anger / Irritability

- Anger aggravated when others didn't listen to me.

[A/f/1,∗/iv]

- Felt a lot of anger and impatience. Was feeling so tense, so restless.

[A/f/1,∗/iv]

- Got very angry and panicky when a friend lost an important paper. Became rude, loud, aggressive, shouted in my anger. "How can they talk to me this way?" Clenched my fists and jaws in anger. Felt I could do anything in anger, even hit someone.

[A/f/1,∗/iv]

- Wanted to lie down. Anger ameliorated by lying down.

[A/f/1,∗/iv]

- Anger – uncontrollable. Felt I could burst out at anyone. Once snapped at a professor.

[A/f/1,∗/iv]

- Irritability, but unable to express it.

[A/f/2,∗/iv]

- Impatience. Felt friend was writing too slowly. Was getting irritated and anxious. Wanted to clutch something with my hands, or tear the paper. Had to control my anger and irritability.

[A/f/2,∗/iv]

- Anger, rudeness on being interrupted, was "wild".

[A/f/2,∗/iv]

- Do not care about the surroundings when I am angry. I curse or snap in public, or in the presence of other family members.

[B/f/2,∗/iv]

- Was irritable at trifles.

[C/m/2,∗/iv]

- Have been getting very angry, and giving people hostile looks.

[D/f/1,∗/iv]

- Angry when co-passenger in a crowded local train complained when I stepped on her foot. Stared at her in anger and confronted her; felt "Couldn't she see how uncomfortable I was!"

[A/f/2,∗/iv]

- I had to attend a community lunch at the temple, where the food was served after a very long delay. While it was being served, there were repeated announcements asking everyone to eat less. This made me very angry and I spoke in an unusually loud tone for a public place. I felt that they were treating us like beggars, as if we were attending it out of our own need. I decided never to attend religious functions henceforth, and left the place without eating.

[B/f/2,∗/iv]

Quarrelsome

- People complained that I was dangerous. Was scolding and quarrelsome with servants, threatened them: "Either you do this or I will stop payments!"
  [D/f/1,*/iv]

- Quarrelsome, sulking, irritable.
  [B/f/2,*/iv]

Suspicious / Mistrustful

- Suspicious – felt that people were saying bad things about me.
  [D/f/1,*/iv]

- Hid money away from my father fearing he would squander it. Didn't trust him.
  [D/f/1,*/iv]

Malice

- Malicious intent, though appear calm outside.
  [D/f/1,*/iv]

- Felt that when others wanted something from me, they were being nice to me. Decided that if people were good to me. I would be the same with them, but if they hurt me, I would be their worst enemy.
  [D/f/1,*/iv]

Restlessness

- A lot of anxiety and restlessness. Unable to sit in one place. If I control my anxiety and sit, I feel tired.
  [A/f/1,*/iv]

- Restless, anxious aggravated between 4 p.m. and 8 p.m. Was unable to sit in one place.
  [B/f/1,*/iv]

- Restlessness ameliorated in the open air.
  [B/f/1,*/iv]

Sadness

- Depression and anxiety in the chest; sort of "doomed down".
  [C/m/2,*/iv]

- Sadness and weeping with headache.
  [A/f/1,*/iv]

- Felt lonely. Was missing my family. Wanted to go home. Felt like weeping and weeping.
  [A/f/1,*/iv]

Green

- Had a liking for green coloured clothes.
  [A/f/*,*/iv]

- Preference for green colour.
  [B/f/*,*/iv]

- Preference for green coloured clothes.
  [C/m/*,*/iv]

- Was excited and fascinated seeing a voluptuous woman wearing a bright, green dress and snake-like ear rings. Was fascinated with her eyes which looked dangerous.
  [D/f/1,*/iv]

Miscellaneous

- While travelling in a crowded train was made uncomfortable by a fellow passenger. Retorted in a commanding yet modest way. Thought I should write a book on how to stand at the door in a Bombay train, so that six people can stand comfortably in a very small space.
  [C/m/2,*/iv]

- Complaining.
  [A/f/2,*/iv]

- Others noticed that I had become contemptuous and was acting superior. Was deliberately using complicated words which people wouldn't understand, and was getting a lot of satisfaction when they would ask me for an explanation.
  [D/f/1,*/iv]

- Had become censorious and snappish. Self-righteously argued with a friend, and held my point till I was disproved.
  [D/f/1,*/iv]

- Better in company, worse when alone.
  [A/f/1,*/iv]

- Aversion to company with the headache.

[A/f/1,*/iv]

- Anxiety for sick brother increased to a horrible degree.

[B/f/1,*/iv]

- Anxiety for family members, ameliorated from being occupied.

[B/f/1,*/iv]

- Wanted to talk to a friend and tell her how much I appreciate her, like her and care for her. But couldn't get myself to do it.

[A/f/1,*/iv]

- Felt I didn't care too much anymore about what others feel about me.

[C/m/2,*/iv]

- Couldn't tolerate noise with the headache.

[A/f/1,*/iv]

- Aversion to music.

[A/f/1,*/iv]

- Felt that a lot of people had a resemblance to my acquaintances.

[C/m/1,2/iv]

DREAMS

Guest

- We were in a small, narrow house with one room and a kitchen, and were asked to sleep on the kitchen shelves. Soon, some more people entered the kitchen saying that this was their usual sleeping place every night. Our host sent them away saying that she had guests, and so there was no room for them. They left, but I felt sorry for them. Then I advised my sister against sleeping on a tall, narrow shelf as she may fall off. On one of the shelves, there was a woman sleeping. On seeing us, she got up, aplogized and left.

Then I was called by my mother to work. It was already morning, and it was no use sleeping now. I felt I had spent all night searching for a place to sleep. I felt bad for the people who slept there every night.

[A/f/2,*/iv]

- A guest is frying fish in our kitchen. I don't like it because we are vegetarian Jains [1]. I am also fearful that my mother-in-law will find out and scold me. But I feel I have to

---

[1] Indian community with austere religious practices.

bear it because the person is a guest – I cannot ask him to stop.

[B/f/1,*/iv]

- One of my friends comes to stay over. He becomes gloomy and wants to be by himself. Then he suddenly appears in the room where I am sitting with my parents, wearing only orange underpants, with white stripes. He is not ashamed that my parents are present.

[About my friend: He has a good name in society and is conscious that he shouldn't do anything that will make him an outcaste. He will not do what is not normal in society. He is timid, careful that he is not criticized, and feels inferior about himself. Such behaviour (appearing in his underpants) would not be expected from him.]

[C/m/1,1/i]

Sexuality

- My aunt is wearing a dress. I insist she wear a saree instead, saying that it will look good on her. My intentions are seductive. She changes into a saree and I admire her figure. Then I ask her to change into another saree. As she goes to change, I follow her and start playing with her sexually. Following the dream I had a nocturnal emission.

[C/m/1,4/iv]

- Two boys fall in love with girls, and others know about it.

[C/m/2,*/iv]

- I had gone for a cruise by myself. The boat was very deep; one half of it was covered from above and the other half was open, so that we had to jump inside. There were many pretty girls with me and I tried to attract their attention. There were many holes in the boat, and it eventually upturned. No one seemed afraid; they jumped out and swam ashore. There were colourful flowers on the land, and everyone else went to see the landscape. I decided to go for a swim. The water seemed shallow. I plunged into it and felt peaceful in the glitter of the sun. Later I felt a bit scared as to what might happen if the water got deeper. I struck the water with my hand, and a black figure with pink lips held my hand and tried to kiss me.

[C/m/1,*/iv]

- Three or four rabbits, coloured pink and fluorescent green, were in a forest. Suddenly, some men appeared to catch the rabbits. All the rabbits ran in a direction away from the men, except for one which was running in the direction towards the men. A goat appeared and advised the rabbit against running in that direction, but the rabbit did not take heed. It ran after a beautiful girl. One of the men caught the rabbit, put it into a bag, and took it to the city.

[B/f/1,*/iv]

- Holi[1]

[B/f/1,*/iv]

---

[1]   A very popular Indian festival when people throw coloured water on each other. Men use this opportunity to take liberties with women, which are otherwise prohibited in Indian society.

- A girl invites a movie actor to her home to have sex. They make love in the rain, and this is broadcast on television. I am watching this in the presence of my family members and am not ashamed. In fact, I am enjoying it and feel aroused. I suggest to my wife that we go and do the same thing under the shower.

Fruits / Vegetables

- Ripe vegetables and fruits in the fridge.

[B/f/1,*/iv]

- A lorry filled with apples is going along a road. There is snow all around. There are film stars and models present. It seems as if we are in Kashmir [2].

[B/f/2,*/iv]

Courts / Trials / Police

- Judicial court.

[B/f/1,*/iv]

- Trial of a film actress.

[B/f/1,*/iv]

- My uncle conducts a trial of his older brother and sentences him to execution. He is being taken in a procession. A coconut is broken. I wanted to help him – feel helpless and sad.

[E'/m/*,*/0]

- Anti-social elements and police.

[B/f/1,*/iv]

- Being pursued by the police.

[B/f/1,*/iv]

- A lock-up with a half open gate.

[B/f/2,*/iv]

Deceit

- My wife disclosed to me, after we were married that she had epilepsy. She was embarrassed to tell me about it. It had been an arranged marriage. I had to either accept her or reject her. She was mild, and depended on my mercy. I accepted her, but felt cheated.

---

[2]   Beautiful, mountainous, northern Indian state.

The thought came to me that they had "made a goat of me" [1] by keeping the matter a secret until after we were married. I tried to tell myself that she could have developed it even after we were married, but accepted the idea with much reluctance.

[E'/m/*,*/0]

• I was watching a movie in which the actor was playing a double role. He was trying to hide his double from the villain. Then there was a funeral pyre with the body of the hero. Somehow, his head had been replaced so that the villain wouldn't know it was the body of the hero. I came to know through someone that the film was called MMM.

[C/m/1,4/iv]

Friends

• I was joining college along with two very close friends. The woman in charge of admissions readily gave us forms which consisted merely of narrow strips of paper. I was puzzled as to how to fill them. I was very glad to be with my close friends again, and wanted that we should be together.

[A/f/2,*/iv]

• Old friends.

[B/f/1,*/iv]

• Old friends.

[C/m/2,*/iv]

Fear

• A villager is fishing with a hook. He is able to catch fish at the first try. My husband suggested that we go into the water for a swim, but I am afraid of drowning.

[B/f/1,*/iv]

• My husband was teaching me to drive a car. Suddenly, something came in the way, and he was asking me to apply the brakes. I was unable to find them, and was fearful of

meeting with an accident.

[B/f/1,*/iv]

Miscellaneous

• My friend is standing on a patch of grassy land which was bright green.

[E'/m/*,*/0]

• I was arguing angrily with friends. My husband felt irritated because I am angry.

[B/f/2,*/iv]

• One of my (dead) teachers was guiding me whilst I was searching for my friend in the market. When I expressed surprise at his being alive, he asked me to touch him so that I would be convinced. I could feel him when I did so.

[B/f/1,*/iv]

• A yogic [2] process is on in which one has to do something with a sharp stick and green peas.

[B/f/1,*/iv]

• A temple being renovated.

[B/f/1,*/iv]

• A man asks my husband and me for a lift. He then invites us home and introduces us to his wife who is elder than him.

[B/f/1,*/iv]

• I bargain over a book with a bookseller, but do not buy it.

[B/f/1,*/iv]

• My brother struck his head against the wall. He had a big ecchymotic patch on the frontal region. I was afraid he would die.

[B/f/1,*/iv]

• I was visited by a female patient who was expecting her second child, and had a high blood pressure.

[B/f/2,*/iv]

• I am in a telephone conversation with a friend, when the receiver starts becoming larger so that I cannot hold it anymore.

[B/f/2,*/iv]

---

[1]   "To make a goat of" is a common Indian expression which implies that since I was non protesting, I was made a sacrificial animal.

[2]   Yoga: Ancient Hindu philosophy.

- I found insects and cockroaches in my pants, and thought to myself that my maidservant doesn't wash my clothes properly.
  [B/f/2,*/iv]

- I try to break open a vial of medicine, and the contents spill out.
  [B/f/2,*/iv]

- Preferring to stay away from home.
  [C/m/1,*/iv]

- I was told by the master prover that the name of the drug being proved was "Thera". It was a known drug and when it had been proved earlier in a higher potency, the provers had developed a severe chest pain which was aggravated at 7.45 p.m. I confirmed the modality of aggravation during the proving.
  [C/f/1,2/ii]

- Too many dreams – felt the night had been too long.
  [E'/m/*,*/0]

PHYSICAL SYMPTOMS

Generalities

- Desire cold tea.
  [A/f/1,*/iv]

- Desire cold milk.
  [A/f/1,*/iv]

- Desire cold bathing; couldn't tolerate even lukewarm bathing.
  [A/f/1,*/iv]

- Aversion to coverings.
  [A/f/1,*/iv]

- Desires sweets.
  [B/f/1,1/i]

- Desires fried food.
  [B/f/1,*/iv]

- Desire spicy food.
  [B/f/1,*/iv]

- Energetic, despite working all day.
  [B/f/2,*/iv]

- Pain left side of the body.
  [B/f/2,*/iv]

- Aggravated by, and unable to tolerate heat.
  [C/m/1,2/ii]

Particulars symptoms

Vertigo

- Felt all things were moving. Had to hold my head, with both hands in order to visualize an object properly.
  [B/f/1,*/iv]

Head

- Headpain – severe : left-sided; frontal, temporal; aggravated between 12.00 noon and 7.00 p.m.; ameliorated from sleep.
  [A/f/1,*/iv]

- Congestive headache in frontal region.
  [B/f/1,*/iv]

- Heaviness in the vertex, aggravated from exposure to sun, aggravated from slightest motion of the head. Unable to keep the eyes open or to read. Blinking and sneezing

with headache.
[B/f/1,∗/iv]

▪ Heaviness over both the eyes, ameliorated by pulling hair.
[B/f/1,∗/iv]

▪ Pain in occipital region.
[B/f/1,∗/iv]

▪ Head pain between 10.00 a.m. and 3.00 p.m.
[B/f/1,∗/iv]

▪ Pain – left side of head.
[B/f/2,∗/iv]

▪ Head pain, on waking in the morning.
[E'/m/∗,∗/0]

Eyes
▪ Blinking.
[B/f/1,∗/iv]

▪ Pain in both eyes on waking.
[E'/m/∗,∗/0]

Nose
▪ Sneezing.
[B/f/1,∗/iv]

▪ Pain, root of nose.
[B/f/2,∗/iv]

▪ Acute sense of smell.
[B/f/2,∗/iv]

Stomach
▪ Appetite decreased, unable to eat from anxiety.
[B/f/1,∗/iv]

▪ Burning in the epigastrium not relieved by cold water. Aggravated after eating. Ameliorated from bending double.
[B/f/2,∗/iv]

▪ Thirst increased.
[C/m/1,2/ii]

Abdomen
▪ Heaviness in the abdomen as from a mass.
[B/f/2,∗/iv]

Stool
▪ Usual constipation was ameliorated.
[B/f/1,∗/iv]

Kidneys, Bladder, Micturation
▪ Urine hot and burning.
[B/f/2,∗/iv]

Male genitalia
▪ Nocturnal emission with amorous dream.
[C/m/1,4/ii]

Female genitalia
▪ Menses too scanty, but had the sensation as if too much blood was passing out through the vagina.
[B/f/1,∗/iv]

▪ Leucorrhoea, curd-like.
[B/f/2,∗/iv]

Voice
▪ Heaviness of voice.
[B/f/1,2/iv]

Chest
▪ Anxiety felt in chest.
[C/m/2,∗/iv]

Back
▪ Sharp pain" like hell" in between the scapulae, with much stiffness in region of neck, and restricted movements.
[B/f/1,∗/iv]

Extremities
▪ Pain in the flexors of the left thigh.
[B/f/2,∗/iv]

Sleep
▪ Waking unrefreshed.
[E'/m/∗,∗/0]

RUBRICS

Mind

Single symptoms

— Anger, clutch someone, impulse to.
— Anger, lying down ameliorates.
— Anxiety, family, about his, ameliorated, occupation, from.
— **Colour, desires green**.
— Delusion, talking ill about him, people are.
— Dreams, advice not heeding.
— Dreams, amorous, having sex in the rain.
— Dreams, animals, rabbits.
— Dreams, anti-social elements.
— Dreams, arguments with friends.
— Dreams, bed, narrow, too.
— Dreams, bed, she had to hunt all night for a place to sleep.
— Dreams, brakes, cannot find while driving.
— Dreams, caught, being.
— Dreams, courts, judicial.
— Dreams, deceit.
— Dreams, deceived, of being.
— Dreams, drowning, fear of.
— Dreams, girls, pretty.
— Dreams, girls, running after a.
— Dreams, girls, trying to attract the attention of.
— Dreams, green meadows.
— **Dreams, guests.**
— Dreams, guests, deprived of their bed by guests.
— *Dreams, guests, unable to ask a guest to stop what he is doing*.

— Dreams, insects and cockroaches in her pants.
— Dreams, kissed, he was, by a black figure with pink lips.
— Dreams, lock-up with half-open gate.
— Dreams, sexual activity being broadcast on television.
— Dreams, sexual play with aunt.
— *Dreams, shameless being*.
— Dreams, shameless behaviour, guest, of.
— *Indifference, others around him, to*.
— Indifference, opinion of others, to.
— Restlessness, anxious, afternoon 4 p.m. until 11 p.m.
— Sadness, melancholy, doomed down, as if.

Common symptoms

— *Anger, irascibility*.
— Anger, morning, waking, on.
— **Anger, easily**.
— Anger, interruption from.
— *Anger, trifles, at*.
— *Anger, uncontrollable*.
— Answers, snappishly.
— Anxiety, chest, in.
— Censorious.
— Complaining.
— Company, desire for, alone, when, aggravates.
— Company, aversion to, head pain, with.
— Contemptuous.
— *Dreams, amorous*.
— Dreams, amorous, pollutions, with.

— Dreams, animals.
— Dreams, animals, goat.
— Dreams, anxious.
— Dreams, flowers.
— *Dreams, friends, old.*
— Drems, fruits.
— Dreams, lascivious.
— Dreams, pursued.
— Dreams, quarrels.
— Dreams, vegetables.
— Home, desires to go.
— Homesickness.
— *Hurry, haste, everybody moves too slowly.*
— Impatience.
— Indignation.
— Indolence, aversion to work.
— *Irritability.*
— *Irritability, trifles, from.*
— Malicious.
— Music, aversion to.
— *Quarrelsomeness, scolding.*
— Rage, fury.

— *Restlessness, nervousness.*
— Restlessness, air, open ameliorates.
— Restlessness, anxious.
— Restlessness, driving from place to place.
— Restlessness, move, must constantly.
— Rudeness.
— Sadness, melancholy.
— Sadness, melancholy, headache, during.
— Sadness, melancholy, weeping, with.
— Sensitive, oversensitive.
— Sensitive, oversensitive, noise, to.
— Sensitive, oversensitive, odours, to.
— *Shrieking, screaming, shouting, anger, during.*
— Striking, desire to strike.
— Sulking.
— Suspicious, mistrustful.
— Threatening.
— Weeping, tearful mood.
— Weeping, tearful mood, headache, with.

Physical symptoms

Generalities
– Bathing, cold bathing, desire for, with intolerance for warm bathing.
– Covers, aversion to.
– Food and drink, fried food: desires.
– Food and drink, milk: desires, cold.
– Food and drink, spices: desires.
– Food and drink, sweets: desires.
– Food and drink, tea: desires, cold.
– Pain, left side of the body.
– Strength, sensation of.
– Warmth aggravates.

Vertigo
– Objects turn in a circle, seem to, room whirls.
– Turning, everything were turning in a circle, as if.

Head
– Fullness, forehead, in.
– Heaviness, forehead, eyes, above, pulling hair ameliorates.
– *Pain.*
– Pain, morning, waking, o·
– Pain, morning, 10 a.m. ⏝ p.m., until.

- Pain, accompanied by eye-blinking.
- Pain, accompanied by sneezing.
- Pain, close eyes, compelled to.
- Pain, pulling hair ameliorates.
- Pain, forehead, left side.
- Pain, forehead noon, 7.00 p.m., until.
- Pain, forehead, sleep, after, ameliorates.
- Pain, occiput.
- Pain, temples, left.
- Pain, temples, noon, 7.00 p.m. ameliorates.
- Pain, temples, sleep, after, ameliorates.
- Pain, pressing, vertex, in.
- Pain, pressing, vertex, motion, slightest aggravates.
- Pain, pressing, vertex, sun from exposure to.

Eyes
- Pain, morning, waking.
- Winking.

Nose
- Pain, root.
- Smell, acute.
- Sneezing.

Stomach
- Appetite diminished, anxiety, from.

- Pain, burning, bending double ameliorates.
- Pain, burning, eating, after.

Abdomen
- Heaviness.

Urine
- Burning.
- Hot.

Male genitalia / Sex
- Pollutions, night dreams, with.

Female genitalia
- Leucorrhoea, curdy.
- Menses, scanty, profuse flow, with sensation of.

Larynx
- Voice, hoarseness.

Chest
- Anxiety, in.

Back
- Pain, scapulae, between.
- Stiffness, cervical region.

Extremities
- Pain, thigh left.

Sleep
- Unrefreshing.

THEMES

1. **Anger**
   Rude.
   Loud.
   Aggressive.
   Shouting.
   Clutch someone, desire to.
   Things not according to her will, when.
   Snapping at professor.
   When made uncomfortable.
   In spite of public place/family members.
   Being made to wait for lunch and then asked to eat less. Felt treated like a beggar.
   Trifles, at.
   Impatience, snapping,

2. Restlessness.

3. **Guest**
   Unable to stop a guest from frying fish.
   Guests taking up their sleeping space.
   Guest appearing in his underwear.

4. **Crowded together**
   At community lunch.
   Sleeping on kitchen shelves.
   Trains.

5. Wanting to be with old friends.

6. **Fears**
   Drowning.
   Accident.

7. **Shamelessness**
   Sex broadcast on TV.
   Friend who stayed over at his house appearing in underpants in the presence of parents.

8. **Sexual**
   Rabbit chasing a beautiful girl, against advise.
   Kissed by a figure with pink lips.
   Attracting pretty girls.
   Sexual play with aunt.
   Holi.

9. **Police, anti-social elements, courts**
   Lock-up with half-open gate.
   Criminal being deceitful.
   Deceived into marrying epileptic woman.

10. Guided by dead teacher.

11. Fruits, vegetables.

12. Green, pastures, green clothes.

13. Lonely, feeling.

14. Quarrelsome, irritable, scolding.

15. Malicious.

16. Threatening, hostile.

17. Contemptuous, superior, critical.

18. Suspicious.

5

A PROVING OF *LAC DEFLORATUM*

A short dream-proving of *Lac defloratum* in the 30 C and 200 C potency, was conducted with thirteen persons, including myself. The provers were between the ages of twenty-three and thirty-four years.

Participants were given one powder in 30 C potency, and instructed to note down their dreams. Prover M did not take the dose. Nobody except the person who selected the drug knew what was being proved. After one week, the proving was discussed, participants were told the name of the drug, and given one powder in the 200 C potency to study the proving effects further.

The potencies were obtained from "Roy and Company", Bombay.

DREAMS

Beaten

- I am carrying something very dirty in a bag to throw it off. But I have both my hands full. So I keep the bag on my head, and all the dirt falls out on my head.

Then I am standing with my sisters and mother in front of the shop we own. It is Diwali [1] and it is brightly lit everywhere. Suddenly a car appears at great speed and stops near to where we are. I feel as if something bad is about to happen. Three women and two men hastily get out of the car and start to beat up an obese. elderly woman who was walking past. They beat her mercilessly and tear off her clothes, and also the clothes of another woman. Everyone around is simply watching them. I am screaming and crying almost hysterically, pleading to my mother to let me go and help them. But I am not allowed to. As these people leave, they look towards us. Their faces are absolutely emotionless and robot-like. I am trying to note the registration number of their car: it is very complicated and in the form of equations (i.e. 9-2/8-9C).

Then I am on a picnic with my family. I see a temple. Suddenly I see my boyfriend there. He is dressed casually. I ask him what he is doing there, and he replies that he is getting married. There are no emotions on his face. I am shocked to hear this. When I see the bride-to-be I am shocked still further: she is very dark, ugly and the typical "rural

---

*   Hindu festival of lights.

type". I wonder how he is ready to marry her. None of their family members are there. So I wait to attend the function.

Suddenly I see the same car again. So I follow it to note down the registration number. As I am noting it down, another car comes up with great speed and halts near me. The same people get out of it. I am very scared but I have a bottle of shampoo with me and I think that I will throw this into their eyes if they come any nearer to me. One of the men also removes a bottle. At first I think that it is a soda-water bottle which he might hurl at me. My second thought is that it is acid. It is thrown at me and it falls on my body, but I don't feel any pain.

[D/f]

- An animal held upside down by the legs, and being beaten with sticks.

[M'/m]

Helplessness

- I am on a motorcycle together with my boyfriend. He is in the driver's seat. He suddenly takes a turn and starts to go fast. I almost fall off the speeding bike and am trying to sit up again. I feel a sudden fear, and as if there is a heavy weight on my chest. My boyfriend is talking to me, unaware of my plight. I want to tell him to drive slowly but I don't get a chance to do so. He keeps on driving fast. Woke up from this dream very, very scared.

[J/f]

▪ I am travelling in a very crowded bus. At one stop, the conductor rings the bell without looking to the entrance. An old man who is trying to board the bus stumbles on the stairs as his dhoti[1] is stuck in the stairway. He is being pulled along all the way. Together with the other passengers, I start to scream at the driver to stop the bus. I also begin to argue with the bus conductor but the other passengers keep their mouths shut.

[J/f]

▪ I am sitting in the out-patient clinic and the water pipe suddenly starts leaking. Everybody present starts laughing. I am trying my best to shut it off but nobody helps me.

[G/f]

Alone / Neglected / Left out

▪ I take my relatives to the school I had attended as a child. I want to show them the paintings exhibited in the hall, some of which had been done by me in my schooldays. There I realize that a school reunion is going on, for which I have not been invited. Just then I hear two boys passing comments while looking at me. I get very "bugged", go to one of them and threaten him very angrily to repeat what he had just said. He tries to act smart, so I repeat the threat. I am so angry that had he repeated it, I would have smashed him. By this time, the person is frightened and denies having made the comment. Instead he points at the other boy, saying that he was the one who had said it. Then I begin to weep and simultaneously complain to the organizer that I had not been invited to the reunion, along with two or three other ex-students.

[E/m]

▪ I am with the other provers at a gathering to discuss our proving symptoms. I have to go out for few minutes. When I return,

---

[1]   A large piece of cloth draped around the lower part of the body by Indian men.

each of the provers has finished narrating his symptoms, and the master prover has concluded the proving. I tell them all that I have not reported my proving, but nobody listens to me.

[I/f]

▪ A group of us are sitting in a hospital ward on New Year's Day. One of my friends enters and wishes everybody present except me. I feel very bad about it.

[G/f]

▪ I am in our medical shop with my father. There are many customers but none of our assistants is around. I get angry at my father as to how he could send away all the assistants, and shout at him.

[F/m]

Children / Adoption

▪ I enter a shop and see a lot of books on the book-shelf. There are large volumes on childcraft. They are green in colour.

[A/f]

▪ I am in my classroom attending a lecture. Suddenly in the midst of the lecture, my mother comes into the classroom carrying a bag. She sits down on one of the benches. I ask her why she has come. She says that she has brought me food. I tell her that I am now grown up, and she doesn't have to bring me food. I feel embarrassed as to what my friends will say about this. At the same time, I feel sorry for my mother: she has taken pains so that I don't have to remain hungry. But at the same time, I feel angry towards her.

[C/m]

▪ I am in a municipal hospital. I meet my aunt and her child aged two or three years. She expects me to hold him and kiss him. But the child is so dirty (his nose is running, his clothes are muddy) that I don't feel like touching him. I have to force myself to hold him. Just then another of my aunts arrives and I rush to give the child to her.

[K/f]

▪ My girlfriend and I want to buy a dog. We go to a playground where many dogs are being kept, but are not satisfied with any of the dogs there. I see one dog which looks like a human being, and I say that we do not want a dog which looks like a human being. We approach a puppy which is injured and I say that this is the one which we want to adopt. We adopt the dog.

[H/m]

▪ A girl I had known came to me with a six year old female child, saying that it was mine. I was asking myself whether I should adopt this child.

[M'/m]

Family / Group / Community

▪ A poor woman is trying to sell something in a crowded train compartment. It seems as if she is really pleading to the passengers to buy her wares. I feel she has to work so hard because her entire family is dependent on her.

[I/f]

▪ A Muslim ice-cream vendor was enquiring whether the area he was in was predominantly a muslim one. When he was told that it was, he began to sell his ice-cream there.

Then I saw my cousin who also was an ice-cream vendor, and I began to help him by accompanying him and showing him places where he can sell his ice-creams. I took him home and gave him warm water to wash his feet with. I felt that I should help my community members just as the Muslims help theirs.

[L/m]

▪ My younger brother has died. His body is kept in the drawing room. We don't feel much sorrow. Everybody goes to sleep and I am sleeping alone in the drawing room where the dead body is kept. Three robbers break in. They start to steal things. When I try to prevent them they ask me to shut up. I am made to sit quietly. Just then my dead brother gets up, and throws them all to one side. He asks me not to worry, saying that he would protect us all.

[L/m]

Friends

▪ I see one of my neighbours who is crippled. He is falling frequently, being unable to walk properly. I carry him on my back to his fourth storey apartment.

From the window of his house I notice some violent activity in the neighbouring building. I am informed that a surgeon had operated a boy and after the operation, had showed the part removed to the boy's mother. The woman had slapped the surgeon saying that her son had had no problem. She asked the surgeon why he had operated on the boy at all. After that the violence had begun in the form of stone throwing. A friend of mine went forward to try and save the surgeon who was our friend. I was very frightened, not knowing what to do.

[L/m]

▪ I go to attend the marriage of a school friend. There I see my friends coming towards me in slow motion and I too am moving towards them in the same manner. I feel extremely happy to be meeting with old friends.

[I/f]

▪ A friend has come to my house. He locks himself in the kitchen and tries to commit suicide by inhaling cooking gas. I bang at the door, break it open and pull him out into the open air.

[D/f]

▪ I am on my way to a drama, when I ask one of my friends to accompany me to buy fresh turmeric[1]. The vendor tries to deceive me by charging hundred and fifty rupees for turmeric worth fifteen rupees. I get angry and walk away without buying it. I lose track of

---

[1]   Spice used in Indian cooking

my friend and as I know the venue of the drama, I decide to reach there on my own. I hire a cab but realize that I have dropped my purse at the vendor's. So I go back to retrieve it. The vendor reminds me that I have left my purse there. I find it lying in a nearby ditch, pick it up and suspiciously check whether my money is still in there. Then I realize that I have two tickets to the drama. I regret being late as my friend will have to wait outside the hall because of me. In the cab I read the ticket to confirm the exact time of the drama and realize that it is scheduled for the next day. I go home directly, feeling foolish for not having checked the tickets earlier.

[J/f]

- I see my friend. She has come to the college but I don't want to meet her.

[B/m]

Anger / Retaliation
- I have to go to Bombay suburb. But instead of taking the short route, I take a longer one. My friends are with me. We arrive at a railway station where we are asked to weigh ourselves. My friend and I stand on the weighing machine with all our books and bags. The attendant shouts at us and calls us fools. I angrily tell her not to taunt us, saying that she is good at this only because it is her job, and if she were to ask us anything concerned with our profession, we could show her how good we are.

[D/f]

- The librarian is screaming at me for not sitting quietly in the library. I fight back saying that I am sitting quietly, and that she is unnecessarily shouting at me.

[D/f]

- I am arguing with a teacher who opposes my view that another of my teachers can become one of the pillars of Homoeopathy. She first tries to convince me and then starts abusing me. I get angry and hit hard on the glass table which breaks into pieces. The medicine bottles beneath also get shattered to pieces. My hand is bleeding profusely. I am scared and wonder how I could do such a thing.

[J/f]

Danger
- I am with my sister. We see a river nearby. As we go closer we realize that we are on a very high, rocky mountain, and the river is way down below and is full of spiky rocks. It is night time and I see one or two people swimming in it. I feel like going in the water, but my sister tells me that I am stupid to think of swimming in such dangerous waters.

[D/f]

- I was in a rural house at night time, along with my teacher and his four year old son. We heard some eerie sounds. My teacher narrated to us and incident of some ghost-like sounds coming from a burnt funeral pyre. He then went on to tell us how when alcohol was poured on the pyre, the sounds stopped.

Then I saw myself standing on the first floor of the house along with my teacher's son. My teacher was missing. It was raining and I had some fear. I felt that I should have returned home in the evening itself; I would have been so comfortable there.

[E/m]

- I receive a phone call from a gangster and he orders me to inform my father that some consignment of smuggled goods is due to reach on a particular day, and that my father (being in the customs) should get it released. I get nervous and extremely frightened that if I don't tell my father, these people might harm him. On the other hand, I feel my father has never done such a thing in his life time.

[I/f]

Sexuality
- I saw a woman bathing in the nude. I got an erection, woke up and returned to sleep.

[B/m]

- A close friend came to meet me and said that he had slept with his girlfriend and consequently had had a lot of bleeding.

[E/m]

Miscellaneous

- A shop full of green leather footwear.

[A/f]

- I am designing a dress with different shades of green.

[A/f]

- My father wears my trousers and an old shirt. The shirt is torn, so he removes it. I tell my father that the trousers are crumpled, so he must change them.

[B/m]

- I have to go to see a girl (as a prospective partner for an arranged marriage) with my father. Before going there I comb my hair, ensure that my clothes are proper. The girl's father asks me about my profession, so I tell him everything about it. I am feeling relaxed because in my heart I know I am going to refuse. I don't like the girl and only if I like her will the matter go ahead.

[C/m]

- I am attending the OPD (out-patient department) of one honorary physician. I am called outside and instructed to attend the OPD of another honorary physician which I do not want to do. I run back inside the OPD and lock the door from the inside. I feel that the other honorary doctor might appear and see me through the window. I ask all my friends to surround me so that I am hidden from view, and he is not able to spot me.

[J/f]

- I am surrounded on all sides by tigers. Some of them are lying down while some are standing. I am surprised to find myself in the midst of them suddenly.

[J/f]

- A monk comes to our place to ask for food. I offer her my favourite dish but she says that if she has it, I will have to forsake eating it for the rest of my life. I am not ready for that. So I offer her a toy to which I am equally attached. Then I ask my mother to throw away all toys from the house as the monk has instructed me to do.

[D/f]

- I am having a bath but have forgotten to lock the bathroom door. My sister-in-law opens the door and walks in despite having seen me. I shout at her to go out but she does not listen. I feel intensely embarrassed and hide behind the door.

[D/f]

- I am standing on a very crowded platform of a railway station at the peak hour. One man with bad intentions was trying to tell the people how one has to get into a crowded train. I felt he was trying to be malicious.

[I/f]

- A man tries to get into a very crowded ladies compartment of a train. The train gains speed and the ladies are trying to push him out. I feel sympathetic towards the man because the train is already in motion.

[I/f]

- A stone statue of a king becomes alive.

[M'/m]

EXPERIENCE OF PROVER L DURING THE PROVING

- I was at the Rationing Office; the clerks were sending me from one desk to another. I was very angry. I told my friend: "I will fight with them. I won't suppress myself. I don't want to be tuberculous." I abused them. I thought of what they must be doing to poor, illiterate people who totally depend on their ration.

RUBRICS

Mind

Single symptoms
— Anger, authority, against.
— Dreams, adoption.
— Dreams, adoption, adopting injured dog.
— *Dreams, alone and helpless, of being.*
— *Dreams, anger, authority, against.*
— Dreams, anger, at being shouted at, taunted or abused.
— Dreams, animals, tied and beaten with sticks.
— Dreams, animals, tigers, surrounder by.
— Dreams, attacked, of being.
— Drems, cheated, being.
— Dreams, child, dirty.
— *Dreams, colour, of, green.*
— Dreams, crippled man, he carried on his back.
— Dreams, dressing up, of .
— Dreams, faces, emotionless.
— **Dreams, family and community, efforts to help out**.
— Dreams, friends, attempting to save her friends.
— Dreams, friends, separated from her friend
— Dreams, give up things she had to those she was very attached to.
— Dreams, mother, being cared for by his.
— Dreams, neglected, of being.
— Dreams, neglected she was, by the person responsible for her.
— Dreams, statue coming to life.
— Dreams, woman, obese, elderly, being beaten mercilessly.

Common symptoms
— Abusive, insulting.
— **Dreams, anger**.
— *Dreams, animals.*
— Dreams, animals, wild.
— Dreams, beaten, being.
— *Dreams, danger.*
— Dreams, death, brother, of.
— Dreams, dirt.
— Dreams, disgusting.
— Dreams, embarrassment.
— Dreams, friends, meeting, of.
— Dreams, friends, old.
— **Dreams, frightful**.
— Dreams, hiding from danger.
— Dreams, homesickess.
— Dreams, lewd, lascivious, voluptuous.
— Dreams, mother.
— Dreams, pursued, of being.
— Dreams, robbers.
— Dreams, weddings, of.
— Fight, wants to.

THEMES

The main feelings or themes that emerge are:

1. Being abandoned or forsaken by friends; being neglected by friends and community.

2. To do things for one's friends.

3. A strong community feeling.

4. Mothering.

5. Adoption.

6. Being beaten with sticks.

7. Seeing others of his group being beaten and abused by other people/authority, but being helpless against it.

8. Anger against authority.

9. Embarrassment.

10. Attractiveness.

11. Feeling fat, ugly, dark, dirty.

12. Feeling suppressed, of no importance: having no voice.

13. Sense of fear and danger.

14. Being forced to do things.

15. Violence.

16. Being not cared for by the person who should be caring.

17. Need to not hurt friends/community, to do things which are good for them, helping members of the community.

18. Suicide.

19. Green colour.

6

THE PROVING OF *LAC HUMANUM*

I conducted a proving of *Lac humanum* at my seminar in Bombay, in August 1995. The participants were mailed one dose each, with instructions to take the dose one week before the seminar, and to carefully note their symptoms during the week. The doses were of five categories: four of them contained the drug from different sources, while one category was simply Saccharum lactis (placebo). The provers gave up their observations during the seminar. These were studied, discussed with the provers, and the conclusion of the proving reached.

Category A : *Lac humanum* 30 C; the source was a lactating Dutch woman.
Category B : Saccharum lactis.
Category C : *Lac humanum* 30 C; source: Belgian woman.
Category D : *Lac humanum* 30 C; source: Indian woman.
Category E : *Lac humanum* 6 C; source: Indian woman.

The provers are indicated with numbers, while the alphabet indicates the category of the dose. Where the provers did not remember which remedy was given to them, no alphabet but only a number has been indicated. Since the symptoms are based only on the notes that the provers submitted, and since the proving was unsupervised, a lot of the information, especially regarding the time of onset of the symptoms, is incomplete and has therefore been omitted.

MIND

Emotions

Two wills

- Constant dilemma of being highly spiritual and God fearing, against bouts of being unreligious and sinful – a turmoil. Feel very, very remorseful and guilty after having done something wrong, although while doing it am unable to control myself. Later, also seek the power to control myself, along with repentance.

  [A7/m]

- Persistent thoughts about how to improve my work, while at the same time the idea kept coming to me of being in a five-star hotel, and just watching movies on television.

  [B4/f]

- Obsessed about individuality versus group conformity. In a dilemma whether I should give more importance to my individuality and speak and question freely, or keep quiet like the rest of the group. In the end, I felt I should give more importance to my individuality and its needs (since my motive was to learn) rather than bother about the rest of the group and how they feel.

  [9'/m]

- Felt dull and lazy; wanted to just lie down, not do anything. Wanted to take two or three days off from work. But went to work because of the commitment. I felt I should do something with my time, otherwise I would be repentant in the evening.

  [23/m]

- Don't want to attend group meetings, but go because of commitment, because otherwise I will feel guilty and spoil the rest of my day.

  [24/m]

Alone / Forsaken

- Quarreled with my mother with the feeling of being left out, alone, as if there was no one with me, not even those whom I love very much (when her mother served her food in an odd plate).

  [A'2/f]

- "Isolated" feeling as if no one cares for me, or as if there is no one to look after me. I feel all are busy in their own lives.

  [A25/f]

- Felt very angry at parents for doing something against my wish. Felt I had many times sacrificed my desires for them and had done things against my wishes for them. Wept a lot, feeling as if I was all alone in the world. Pushed away my mother very hard in my anger and told her that I would never eat anything made by her again. After a while was repentant about my behaviour.

  [A28/f]

- Almost in tears with an intense forsaken feeling when my mother gave more food to my brother than to the rest of us. Scolded her saying that she cared for him and didn't love me.

  [A/35/f]

- Angry at husband for returning late; shouted at him, clenched teeth, pounced on him, asked him to kill me because I could no longer bear to live alone waiting for him.

[D7/f]

- Feeling "cut off " from my friends circle; I don't want to be with them, or I am unable to maintain a relationship with them. I feel that if they do not want me, I should leave them alone and be free. I feel like I have done a lot of things for them but they give me nothing in return, that they reject me because I am of no use to them, that they have chosen their path and I must choose mine.

[8'/m]

- Felt as if I was alone, there was no one there for me.

[A20/f]

- "Wild" with anger on friends when they neglected me and sat amongst themselves, although I had reserved seats for them in the seminar. Felt ignored, like I had no value. Felt that people don't understand or consider me although I try to help them in many ways. Felt the need of someone who understands me.

[3/m]

- I felt it is preferable to stay alone and concentrate on your aim, because then you have a position and people appreciate you.

[5/f]

Irritability

- Irritable and excited from trifles.

[A'2/f]

- Irritability.

[A6/m]

- Irritable, rude and hurtful to family members, especially my mother. But would apologize immediately and think about how much my mother has done for me; wanted to spend as much time with my mother as was possible for me.

[A 34/f]

- Tremendous irritability. Desire to be silent, taciturn.

[A 36/f]

- Easily irritable, rebellious, rude in speech and behaviour, back answering and hurtful to those around.

[D13/f]

- Irritable, easily annoyed.

[17/f]

- Irritable, depressed, quarrelsome, with family and friends over trivial matters. Felt they were self-centered.

[3/m]

- Quarrelsome, irritable, especially with family.

[4]

Sadness / Weeping

- Wept with an inability to express what I was feeling.

[A4/f]

- Excessive, causeless weeping.

[A27/f]

- Weeping in the evening at 5 p.m.

[A 20/f]

- Depressed with recollection of sad thoughts.

[A30/f]

- Depressed and dull mood.

[A33/f]

- Weeping everyday at 2 p.m.

[15/f]

- Weeping and tearful often.

[6/f]

Despair

- Had the depressing feeling that I can't do anything bright in the future.

[A25/f]

- Sudden thought that I should die since it is of no use to live.

[A20/f]

- Strongly averse to company. Wanted to be alone to sit or lie down and weep. Felt disgusted, hopeless, good for nothing, as if there was nothing in life to live for; to continue to live is the most painful thing.

[D3/m]

• Feeling, on being scolded, as if people don't care, or as if I am alone. I feel they can't understand me and that I should commit suicide because it does not make a difference whether I live or die.

[6/f]

Impulses

• Had the impulse to run in the corridor and beat someone.

[A29/f]

• Sudden impulse to throttle a teacher, which vanished in a few seconds.

[B3/f]

• Tendency to inflict self-harm; burnt palm, and made a cut with a pen knife.

[C3/f]

Restlessness / Hurry / Impatience

• Impatient and hurried. Too many thoughts came to mind; could not hold on to any thought for long and could not concentrate for long.

[7/m]

• Feeling internally impatient and bored, without wanting to show these feelings to others.

[C1/m]

• Restless, without understanding why.

[A31/m]

• Driving unusually fast, wanted to overtake all other vehicles on the road.

[A31/m]

Work and rest

• No drive or enthusiasm. Feeling that work is routine. Want to do things, have big plans in mind but do not put them into practice. Feel that it is okay if I don't do them.

[30/f]

• Lack of enthusiasm. Content with having nothing done.

[25/m]

• Making plans to study, but doing very little.

[24/m]

• Wanted to take leave, to take a break from work and come back refreshed.

[27/f]

• Wanted a break from work, wasn't happy with myself, wasn't benefiting much from it.

[24/m]

• Feel that I need a break, and that after a break my boredom will go.

[23/m]

• Bored with routine. So went on a picnic. But after that break was feeling that the same routine started.

[28/m]

• Feel the need to work hard.

[24/m]

• Feel enthusiastic. Want to do something new, to start again. Feeling like one has to do something.

[29/m]

• Have the feeling that one shouldn't sit without doing any work, that "rest is the devil".

[D6/f]

• Unsuccessful efforts to finish work "stuck up".

[D6/f]

• Alternate state: hectic activity on the one hand, doing many things in a short time, and lack of enthusiasm on the other.

[28/m]

Miscellaneous

• Indifference to everything around me. Inability to realize my rudeness towards family members. Totally self-oriented.

[D13/f]

• Indifference to my cousin (who I discovered had double-crossed me and was having an affair with my boyfriend). Though depressed over the matter, did not weep bitterly as I would have otherwise done in such a circumstance.

[C3/f]

■ Indifference to all things and feelings.

[C3/f]

■ Lacking in my usual conscientiousness in giving explanations about my behaviour.

[A 39/f]

■ Embarrassed and hiding, thinking what others would say about him when he could not control his urge to eat much and frequently.

[20/m]

■ Very talkative, so that others around me are "bugged".

[A29/f]

■ Desire to be silent.

[A1/m]

■ No desire to talk to others, nor to do anything.

[D1/m]

■ Taciturn. Averse to answering. Answering in monosyllables.

[5/f]

■ Quarrelsome over trivial matters, repentant later.

[A31/m]

■ Tranquility, a kind of quietude in situations where I would have been irritable or flustered.

[A 39/f]

■ Usual anxiety (about profession, finance, etc.) was ameliorated.

[A1/m]

■ Introspection and calmness.

[A1/m]

■ Anxiety about everything.

[15/f]

■ Sudden curling up from fright when accidently touched during sleep.

[B3/f]

■ Desires objects and rejects the same when they are offered.

[C3/f]

■ Loud, dominating speech. Making others do whatever I wanted them to.

[C5/m]

■ Wanted to attract others towards myself.

[D1/m]

■ Many strange thoughts and I don't know what is the real thing.

[D2/m]

■ Desire to walk gracefully.

[D9/f]

■ Decreased confidence in the daytime. Ameliorated in the evening.

[D12/m]

■ Depressed, wept violently from quarrel with brother. Wondered how could he hurt me so easily when I am so nice and caring towards him. I felt that loving somebody only causes you pain. You love your mother, brother, relatives and friends but they care least for you; these relations only cause you pain. I wondered why man creates so many relations, why he wants to live with so many people around him when it only hurts him or depresses him.

[D13/f]

■ Desire to help out my mother.

[A20/f]

■ Felt as if no one cares in the outside world except one's immediate family, only they can understand you and handle your problems. So it is better to remain with them than with friends and other relatives.

[5/f]

■ Sudden memories of an old teacher, with the thought of meeting him and having a nice chat with him.

[2'/f]

■ Feeling as if something needs to be hidden.

[32/m]

Intellect

- Dullness.
  [A1/m]

- Dullness in the evening, around 5.00 p.m.- 6.00 p.m.
  [A3/*]

- Inability to concentrate.
  [A6/m]

- Increased ability to think.
  [A8/m]

- Clarity of mind with increased ability for mental work.
  [A'35/f]

- Sudden confusion of mind as to the day of the week, took sometime to recollect.
  [B3/f]

- Tired and fagged out. Unable to concentrate or exert the mind.
  [D3/m]

- Was thinking about what would happen were human milk to be proved; whether if it was proved from different sources, we would obtain common symptoms pertaining to the state of mind of the individual from whom the substance was collected.
  [21'/m]

DREAMS

Alone / Forsaken / Deserted

- Dreams as if left alone in the wilderness, or as if alone in the world.
  [A1/m]

- Weeping because a friend scolded me for improper behaviour, with the feeling that I was all alone.
  [A'2/f]

- My aunt, to whom I am very close and attached, befriends a woman when we are travelling together in a train. As the train stops at a station along the way, my aunt suddenly asks me to get off. I tell her that I do not know anyone in the place and have nowhere to go. But she throws me out of the train with my luggage, saying that she wants some time alone with her new friend and she will come for me after two or three days. I was left alone at the station, not knowing what to do or where to go. I was very furious but also extremely jealous that inspite of being so close to my aunt, she had deceived me for someone she hardly knew.
  [A 19/f]

- I was alone in a tall building. I was scared to enter the lift because there was no one around, so I took the stairs. While coming down I found myself lost, could not find my way.
  [D 10/f]

- My friends were sitting away from me during an exam. I did not know any answers to the questions asked. I could see my friends discussing answers amongst themselves, but there was no one around to help me. I felt that they would all pass, whilst I would fail and be left alone.
  [D 15/f]

- I was supposed to meet my friend, and we were to go together to the seminar. But I reached a bit late and my friend had left me and gone. I didn't know my way to the seminar, nor did I have enough money to get there by myself.
  [D15/f]

- I was waiting at a bus stand with some friends. We were in a happy mood, singing and joking when the bus came. Some time

118   Provings

later, all my friends ran towards it and got onto it, without paying any attention to me. I was left alone on the bus stand. I felt that there was no one to look after me or care for me. In spite of having done so much for my friends, they didn't understand or care for me, so it was of no use to make friends. I felt that no one thinks for others, and each one thinks only for himself.

[1/m]

▪ I was giving an exam for which I knew all the answers. But while I was writing the paper, a professor came up to me and told me that I was writing "rubbish". He then threw me out of the classroom. I had been writing correctly, and so wondered how he could throw me out. I also had the slight feeling as if I had committed some crime and had been therefore thrown out. But I mainly felt lonely for being the only person who was thrown out, while the rest of the class continued to write the paper. I felt that no one cared for me, that others were selfish and cared only for themselves.

[1/m]

▪ I had organized a picnic with a few friends. We spent the whole day enjoying ourselves; we had our lunch together. As the evening approached, I started to feel depressed. When I looked behind, I found that my friends had disappeared along with all their belongings. I was shocked, lonely, and didn't know what to do.

[3/m]

▪ I go to a seminar in an old hall. I am trying to locate my friends. When I find them, they sit apart from me. I am alone.

In the lunch break we pass through a village-like place, and we are running through it because we are late.

[6/f/, before dose]

▪ While returning from dinner with my friends, I realized that they were not behind me like I had thought. I was left alone.

[6/f]

▪ A criminal was being held by the police. He was wearing a suit with a tomato coloured tie . He had been tied up with a rope which had been wound four times around his body. A policeman was holding the rope tight on one side while I was holding it on the other side. We were trying to pull the criminal in his suit, pant, and neck tie. Just then, somebody told us no matter what we did, he would escape anyway, and that nothing could be done with these people. Suddenly the rope cut open and he escaped.

Suddenly I was on a very empty road with five lanes on either side. I was sitting on a swing with a very long rope coming down as if from the sky. I was swinging and everything was lonely; I felt a sense of utter loneliness, as if I was alone here and there was nothing around. I wondered why criminals or people who trouble others work for just a little money. I also thought about a cousin who is in USA, that he may be working for these kind of people for three thousand dollars. I was very sad and was swinging, tears rolling down from my eyes. There was also the fear that I was alone and those people who were pulling that criminal may get me as well. Suddenly my wife came from behind and asked why I was sitting there. I woke up feeling soothed.

[19'/m]

Helping

▪ My younger cousin brother has an auditory handicap, but he is able to follow lip movements. He is attempting to speak and I am teaching him names of colours: red, yellow and black.

Then I am walking with him on a very quiet street surrounded by trees. I realize that his face is deformed. I see one of my friends who is going to a plastic surgeon for a facelift. I wonder why she needs it. She says she wants to look beautiful. I cannot understand it, but then realize that I too need it for my cousin. So I note down the name and address of the plastic surgeon.

[A 21/f]

- A colleague has been recently married. His previous girlfriend is weeping because he left her alone and married somebody else. I feel bad for this girl and am thinking in what way I can help her.

[A 21/f]

- On a picnic with friends. We were playing mono-acting when a pregnant friend collapsed. We were going to give her a cardiac massage, when a python encircled her abdomen.

[A 25/f]

- Gone on a trekking adventure with friends, to a beautiful place with mountains, rivers and greenery. One of my friends suffered from breathlessness because of the high altitude. I gave him medical assitance and was appreciated by all. While travelling I fought with a porter.

[A 31/m]

- A patient is admitted in status asthmaticus at the hospital where I am working. The honorary doctor in charge starts with the medication, but the patient has no relief. His relatives plead to me to do something, saying that he is dying. I take them to the honorary doctor and inform him of the patient's condition and also that his relatives are asking for a better medicine. He says that he is doing his best and can do nothing more. I feel very helpless and feel were I given the permission to, I would give him the best possible medicine to save his life.

[A 36/f]

- Helping an unknown, sick person, and assuring him that I am fully responsible and would help him back to recovery.

[A 39/f]

- Helping someone in need, out of a sense of duty.

[A 39/f]

- I see a huge crowd outside a building I am driving by. I learn that a very famous film heroine, who is also the wife of my revered teacher, has been murdered by one of her fans. I feel I should go and console my teacher, imagining the intense grief and shock he must be under. Later I realize that the whole thing was only a rumour.

[B1/m]

- I was waiting at a bus stop with an elderly person who was unable to walk properly. I made way for him to climb in, when the bus arrived, but was myself refused entry when I tried to get in. I felt I should think of myself first, and then for others.

[C 5/m]

- I was travelling with my friend. She stopped the car at one spot at the edge of a hill; there were rocks ahead and so the car could not go any further. We got off and began to walk. Suddenly we saw very, very huge animals walking here and there, in comparison to whom we were very small and so they did not notice us. Then a few people came and helped us get the car down again. We drove away quickly as we were a bit scared.

[D 6/f]

- I am living in a hut of which all the doors are wide open. Suddenly I become aware that a Hindu nationalist politician (who had been responsible for Hindu-Muslim riots) is coming to rape my sister and me. He looks like a villain out of a Hindi film. I am "dead scared", and ask my sister to run away with me. Although she asks me not to bother, I take her hand and run. While we are running we come to a house from which a woman calls out to us and on finding out why we are running, she offers us shelter. We hide in her kitchen and I am scared. But I have confidence in this woman although she is a Hindu. Then through the window I see some members of my community (Muslim) who are returning from a religious ceremony. They are surprised to see me here. Then, the daughter of our hostess helps me climb down from the window.

[14'/f]

▪ A doctor friend of mine is arranging vegetables on a railway bridge to sell. I think he has to sell vegetables because he is not doing well in his practice. I ask my son to help him and myself also offer to stand with him to help him sell the vegetables.

[7/m]

▪ A patient, who was paralysed, was lying in a dirty toilet with blood shot eyes. I had to pick him up, support him and take him for a CT scan to a diagnostic centre nearby. The man was very bulky, but I managed to reach him even though I had a tough time doing it.

[16/f]

▪ My friend is to give an exam in the morning, and I too have to appear for an exam the same afternoon. I take my friend to the exam centre and am helping and reassuring her before she goes in. I am fully aware that I am unprepared for my own exam the same afternoon, and myself need to study.

[4'/f]

▪ A man was trying to attack my fellow students, knife them, beat them up. I accosted him alone and gave him a few, good blows. Then I tried to round up my family members, and other people around for help, but somehow, they were not effective enough. So I picked him up twirled him around and threw him down three floors. I thought that would be the end of him, but he managed to break his fall by landing on a passer-by on the street below.

Then I went into a class room and stood against a wall on the teacher's platform, so that I was well protected, in case he came back to attack me. One student objected, but the teacher stuck up for me, saying that I deserved to be protected since I was a brilliant student.

[21/*]

▪ I was visiting the house of my friend's mother. I could hear my friend and her husband from somewhere else in the neighbourhood. Their daughter was in the house and I was told that she had sudden high fever with tiny, red eruptions. I thought of giving her *Belladonna*.

[A4/f]

▪ A senior colleague comes up to a group of us, and hits one of my friends. I get very angry and shout at him for daring to hit her, although no one else says anything.

[A 33/f]

▪ I am alone with an unknown woman who is in labour. I have to conduct the delivery. I am unable, immediately, to suction the baby or sever the umblical cord. I panic that the baby might be dead, but it responds with a cry when I tap it on the back. But I do not sever the umbilical cord at all. On waking I felt I should have severed it.

[A 34/f]

▪ One of my patients gets an aggravation and I have to act fast lest she suffers a lot. I retake her case, get symptoms I have missed, and give her a remedy.

[A 34/f]

▪ My friend and me are playing outside the house and were building castles and houses out of the sand. My father is sitting in the verandah in an easy chair and while we are playing we are grown up somehow. I have to make a payment of some money.

My friend becomes a bank officer and says that he will manage to pass the cheque somehow even though I have no money. I feel my father will scold me for doing such improper things and so I want to conceal it from him. But when the cheque is passed my father somehow finds out and asks me how I could do it. I am angry, almost weeping, and feel I am being wronged, but am unable to tell him anything. The next minute he asks me for some medicine for his throat pain. I feel he has done me wrong, but what can I do; I will give him medicine. I feel he may have done me wrong, but he should get well.

[20/m]

■ My brothers, friends and myself are together on the terrace of a building. We are having fun by shooting at passers-by with arrows made from pencils and broomsticks, with the help of bows. I climb down on a ledge to see how many people are being hit while my friends shoot. I watch with enjoyment and thrill, an old man have his chest and abdomen pierced by three pencils.

I too want to try my aim. I begin to climb an iron ladder that runs from the parapet to the terrace. It is rusted and as I reach its upper half, it gives way. I fall back along with the ladder and am hanging dangerously from the edge of the ledge. I am holding on tightly to the ladder and I can see a drop of many feet below me. I am terribly scared that I may fall any moment. My friends and brothers rush to my help. They use a waterpipe as a fulcrum to bring the ladder up. They are doing it wrong and I want to correct them but am unable to utter a word out of fear. I try to explain through gestures but they do not understand. As they continue to pull me up, a joint in the ladder breaks and I am lowered into the air by about two feet. I am "dead scared", when my brother comes forward and pulls the ladder in the right way so that I am safely back on the parapet.

[A 38/m]

■ I borrow my neighbour's car. I tell him that I will take his car for one hour and I go off. I wander around, loiter, make fun in city. Suddenly I feel like going for a movie. So I drive down and enter into an auditorium. It gets converted into a homoeopathic seminar where the speaker is my friend. I don't know how it happened. The seminar ends in the evening. I get out, not bothered that I had told my neighbour that I would return in one hour.

In the meanwhile, my neighbour starts panicking as to where I have gone. He calls his elder brother, as he usually does in any crisis, and they are discussing where I could have gone with his car. A search party of five persons is out on the street, and suddenly they discover their car lying outside the auditorium. I find all of them sitting around the car when I come out. They ask me why I did not return in one hour like I had told them. I said that I just felt like going for a movie, it got converted into the seminar and I was busy. They were very upset and I distinctly remember the words: "Never ever share the car with anybody." I just felt shameless. It had so happened that I had felt like going off without informing them, I had taken their car, and gone off happily; I felt no sense of shame or guilt.

[19'/m]

■ My sister wakes up and shouts at me for not having woken her up in time for college. She says that henceforth she will not wake me up even if I am getting late. I feel sadness and helplessness, and wonder how I would be able to reach the hospital on time.

[18'/f]

Cousins

■ My cousin and me were unable to get a taxi. After having waited long, I finally managed to get one. But my cousin who had been standing across the street continued to look out for a taxi. I was trying to tell him to cross over since I had already hired one. After a while, when he was unable to get a taxi, he crossed over and sat down beside me in the cab I had kept waiting. I got very irritated and began to shout at him.

[A 20/f]

■ My cousin and my friend had had a fight, and both had died. There were great processions from both the groups.

[A 16/m]

▪ My cousin sister is being killed by a man. The room is full of blood. I try to save her, but her assaulter runs behind me to kill me. I tell a crowd gathered outside my cousin's house of the incident and ask them to save her. I am weeping, and running from the man who is still following me. I am feeling lonely. My life is in danger and I have to escape. The man succeeds in catching me, but I escape, but he begins to pursue me once again. I am frightened.

[A 23/f]

▪ My cousin brother had come to visit me in my hometown. His motorbike was parked outside the house.

[A24/f]

▪ My pregnant cousin goes into labour prematurely. She is in distress and requires assistance. I call for an obstetrician, who conducts a vacuum delivery. The baby is healthy and although its gestational age is only seven months, and his weight is three and a half kilograms. I am fascinated and happy to be playing with the child.

[A 34/f]

▪ My cousin and another woman have just delivered babies in a huge, commercial-looking maternity home that is guarded by policewomen. I admire my cousin's baby who looks better than the other woman's child. It has good features, long length, is quiet, and can be looked after easily. However when it cries, to my surprise its face becomes cyan-osed and resembles the human embryo in the stage where three pairs of pharyngeal arches are present. When it stops crying it resumes its normal form.

[B 3/f]

▪ My cousin is sleeping in the corner room of a house. There are windows on two walls. He suddenly wakes up shouting that there is someone outside the windows. In spite of reassuring him, he doesn't believe me. So I (magically) jump out of one window and open both windows from outside while

floating in the air, and try to convince him.

[D 12/m]

▪ I was in a tunnel-like place, sitting in a corner that was like a trench. I was sitting in front of a gas and teaching my two younger cousins mathematics with a remote control in my hands.

[16/f]

▪ I met a friend while I was going to attend the marriage of my cousin. Her face is scarry, covered with big eruptions. She is upset about her face, and wants to go home. A few minutes later, all the eruptions disappear but she still wants to go home, and so departs. Then I ask my cousin whether she really wants to be married, and she says why not. We are discussing how long we will need to get ready. I see the youngest of my cousins whom I greet. Then I see a very distant cousin who is so emaciated that his shoulder joints are clearly visible. His head has become large and oblong and his eyes are large with blackening beneath them. I call out to him, but he does not listen. I look up and can see my kitchen window, from which broken wooden furniture is hanging out.

[2'/f]

Friends

▪ Death of a friend.

[23/m]

▪ Quarreling with my best friend without knowing why.

[A'2/f]

▪ Being scolded by a friend for having visited the canteen; she was telling me that it was not a wise act.

[A'2/f]

▪ My friends have come to visit and are falsely accusing me of having done some injustice to them. They tell me that I am being watched for an opportunity so that they can punish me.

Later when I go out some unknown

persons are pursuing me and I am returning home.

[A 14/m]

- Some of my friends had hosted a large farewell party for me. As we enjoyed yourselves eating, drinking and laughing, I felt joyous about being together with everyone. I began to collect everyone to join in for a group photograph.

[A15/f]

- Death of a friend.

[D5/m]

- I met with a friend, who was dressed childishly with two pony-tails and was talking funnily.

[D 10/f]

- I was travelling in a car with a group of people. We were all in the nude. I did not recognize any of them as being familiar, but we were all supposed to have been friends. We were going out on a picnic probably to a beach.

On the way another car passed by with another group of people all of whom were also naked. We all waved and shout greetings to each other. I was neither surprised nor embarrassed about being naked or being in the company of naked people. It all seemed okay.

[13/f]

Family / Relatives

- Going out for dinner with my parents who live in another city.

[A'12/m]

- I am waiting at a railway station to receive my near and dear ones. As the train carrying them approaches, its engine derails. Then the engine is knocked off, and the rest of the train continues uncontrolled. It passes onto a railway track which is distorted. I run to a nearby outpost, but no one there seems aware about the uncontrolled train nor about the distorted tracks. I somehow manage to

convince a person in a railway uniform to take some action. He very coolly picks up a telephone and informs the authorities at the next station about the incident.

[A 22/m before dose]

- My father, accompanied by one of our servants, is riding a very unusual looking bicycle with car tyres. I am worried that he may meet with an accident, but he seems unconcerned. I somehow stop him, but ride the bicycle myself.

[A 22/m before dose]

- Relatives.

[A 27/f]

- My uncle who lives in England has come to visit without any prior notice. We are all very much surprised to see him. Then I go to see an aunt whom I have been promising to visit since the last two months.

[A 28/f]

- Praying with father (dead) on a festive occasion. Happy feeling.

[A 32/f]

- My mother (dead) visited me and asked for a drink made from milk. I found it difficult to prepare this, there being not enough milk, and the required vessel being unavailable. But I was happy to prepare it for her.

[A 32/f]

- I am with my relatives on a hill. We are descending with the help of a staircase which is open on one side. The others cross the staircase easily, but with a fear of falling, while I avoid the portion which is open on one side.

[D 12/m]

- I am trying to locate a place, when I see my parents approaching. I ask my father to help me find it, and he guides me. When we are about to part, I notice a large reddish patch of leucoderma on my mother's face, extending across the right side from the forehead almost upto the chin. I am shocked to see it, but my parents walk away before I can say anything.

When I return home, my parents are talking happily. My mother is wearing a bright saree of parrot green and yellow. The skin of her face has almost come back to normal. I anxiously say that she should see a doctor, that the patch is in a very early stage and it will disappear on constitutional treatment. But my parents don't take me seriously and instead make fun of me. All the same I am very anxious and desperate. I bend to write down all her symptoms, and prepare to arrange for an appointment with a homoeopathic physician. I feel that being a doctor this responsibility is mine.

[D 13/f]

▪ Going on a picnic with relatives.

[D 13/f]

Community

▪ I was with many people in a dimly lit house, on a gloomy morning. My mother was getting ready to go to the bank and, as I was helping her with her papers, I noticed a large blood stain on her clothes. I gave her a sanitary napkin and asked her to quickly change.

Then I went outside the house and sat on the stairs with some persons, some of them being my patients. I was mending my nail, when in the garden opposite I saw many saintly people come together. They were all dressed in white, and belonged to various religions. A Muslim woman from amongst them, looked one of my Muslim patients seated next to me, as if to say how could she be sitting next to me (a Hindu). My patient stood up in response to her stare.

[D 7/f]

▪ I was walking with my husband when suddenly riots between Hindus and Muslims broke out. We ran into a neighbouring compound and hid in a railway wagon. I was scared and wanted very much to reach home, but did not dare to come out for fear of being shot. I saw a van full of Muslims, pass by. They were shouting anti-Indian slogans, giving speeches, exciting people against India and urging them to kill other Indians. I was afraid that they might discover us and shoot us.

[A 37]

▪ My brother and me were walking down a road when we heard screams and sounds as if people were pursuing one another, yelling and throwing stones. We realized that there was a Hindu-Muslim riot. My brother suggested that we take another lane which he anticipated might be safer, but we reached there only to find the same situation. We just kept running and running, on and on.

[22'/f]

Journeys / Trains / Roads

▪ Catching a bus.

[30/f]

▪ Travelling in a bus.

[A 24/f]

▪ Going out for a vacation in the snow.

[A 28/f]

▪ On a train journey with a group of college friends and a female teacher. The journey was to be from Bombay to London. We were all happy and excited.

[A 30/m]

▪ My family was about to embark on a journey but were unable to do so since the train was cancelled.

[A/ 32/f]

▪ Trying to get into a crowded local train with a friend, but unable to because of the crowd getting out. We finally do succeed, and I am relieved.

[A'35/f]

▪ I boarded a train. It was going in the opposite direction. So I got off the running train.

[D 10/f]

▪ Was driving along a curved road with friends. There was greenery around. We were all going on a picnic.

- We were driving in a car at high speed on a curved road.

[11/f]

- I arrive at Bombay Central station and find that it looks like a village. Suddenly a new coach train arrived and I saw that it had the names of two trains on it. I was surprised to see that one of them was a train that does not travel to Bombay. I entered the train and it started suddenly. There were very few passengers on board. I met with a person who tried to pull me, but I fought with him.

[A1/m]

- Travelling a deserted road on a scooter, which though straight, had many ups and downs.

[A1/m]

- Driving zig-zag.

[26/m]

Snakes

- I was travelling in a train. It fell off the tracks. I jumped out from the compartment and found myself surrounded by snakes from whom I was trying to escape.

[A'12/m]

- Our entire family has gathered in our old house. One of the members sees an insect, but someone else says that it is a snake. Then we see a small, tiny golden snake about six centimetres long. Everyone is afraid, but I remind them that it is very small, and that besides it is a symbol of God. I want to hold it, but as I approach, it melts into a golden fluid.

[D'11/m]

- A snake wound itself around me while I was travelling in a train. I wasn't scared, picked it up and threw it out, although it was slippery.

[5/f]

- I am in my old house where we lived as a joint family. There is a snake being killed. My sister-in-law asks me why they are killing the snake. I replied that it is very poisonous,

and has to be killed. Suddenly, the snake is on my sister-in-law. Everybody is dumbfounded. I ask everyone not to worry, not to move or do anything, and am repeatedly saying that I will handle the problem and that everything is okay. But my sister-in-law loses patience, and brushes the snake away. Suddenly the snake is converted into a semi-solid chutney-like (sauce/dip) substance, which spills. Everybody is looking to see where it disappeared, when suddenly I realize that it is on my head. I touch my head, and all of a sudden, my right nostril begins to run. The discharge is bluish, like copper sulphate, and very acrid. In a short while, my breathing starts to get very heavy and strenuous. I tell my wife not to worry, that I will get well, though I know I am being poisoned. I ask her to note down all my symptoms, mention everything that I am suffering, because I feel they may be of the snake poisoning. I again assure her that I will be well.

Then my breathing gets even heavier, and when I am hardly able to breathe, I go to my father's dispensary and tell him what is happening to me. I feel he will save me. I awoke breathing heavy, and relieved that it had been a dream.

[19'/m]

- Of being at a party where she had a snake in her bag. The snake is somehow let loose; it is enjoyable for her. But fearing that other people will be bitten, she puts it back into her bag.

[27/f]

Animals

- While roaming in a forest I saw wild animals like snakes, lions and panthers roaming about, and felt no fear.

[A 25/f]

- Two fish in green coloured water.

[D 15/f]

- A big, white cat had entered my house and was trying to destroy it. I caught hold of the cat to remove it from my house, but it slipped out from my hands. I ran after it, caught it and threw it out from the window. In the bargain, I hurt my palm.

[D 15/f]

- I am standing with my classmates at a seashore which is on the terrace of a building. There are numerous rats coming out of the sea, and my classmates are admiring them.

[E 2/f]

- A cat or a cheetah.

[6/f]

- I was on a mountain covered with snow. There was also an animal there.

[11/f]

Floods

- Came out of a big haveli-like building to find water everywhere. I tried to see roads but they were blocked. I informed other people in the building that they had better stay indoors, the roads being blocked.

[A1/m]

- The river of a nearby village had been flooded so that water overflowed from the bridge. My friend and I attempted to cross it even though we knew it was dangerous. To my surprise, the bridge was curtained from both sides. My friend advised that I should not allow the engine to stop otherwise it would not restart because of the water. We managed to reach the other side with some difficulty.

[A1/m]

- Many dreams of heavy rains and floods.

[A1/m]

- Paying a social call, accompanied by my family, on a raft because every street in town is flooded.

[A10/m]

Fearful / Anxious

- Fearful dreams of horror movies.

[A1/m]

- Anxious dreams.

[A1/m]

- Dreams of horrible faces.

[A1/m]

- Fearful.

[A 2/m/ before dose]

- I was trying to remove a block in the needle of a syringe by blowing in air and sucking it out. In the process, I accidently swallowed the needle and I was frightened that it would perforate through my stomach. I imagined the needle piercing through my stomach wall and the fear kept increasing in my mind. I did not know what to do and was afraid that I would die.

[A 38/m]

- Tremendously anxious and hurried about finding a remedy for a patient.

[B 3/f]

Danger

- Everything around me is burning, and I am shouting for help.

[A 27/f]

- Vivid dream of travelling in a bus with familiar people, when suddenly its speed becomes very fast and we reach the edge of a cliff. Down below is a marsh and a turbulent river. We are all screaming and I feel with great fear that this is death. Then my fear is replaced by an acceptance but there is a hope that somehow the driver may be able to help. Suddenly the disaster is averted and we rejoice in our safety. I am immensely relieved and happy. Then surprisingly, we begin to eat corn cobs on which there were big ants crawling, after having brushed them aside.

[A 39/f/before dose]

- Being choked or strangulated.

[E 3/f]

- I was driving very fast while travelling to another city, when a truck appeared before me. But I made no attempt to control my vehicle, nor to give way to the truck. I woke, shaken up, panting, breathless.

[15/f]

■ A friend and me are standing amongst heaps of junk. We look up and see a chemical factory that is so huge that we cannot even see the sky. It is all very colourful.

Then someone comes in a car to kill us, and my friend and me both get into my car, but it will not go ahead, no matter how much I try. So I have to drive very fast in the reverse gear.

[A 33/f]

Pursued

■ My friend and me are being followed and, teased by two or three males.

[A 36/f]

■ I was being pursued by an elephant in the street of my village. I want to hide in the side of the lane but the mahout asks me to go away. I flee, but from a distance I can see the elephant searching, using his trunk. I go to my old home and hide there. When I come out I do not find the elephant, even on much searching.

[10'/m]

■ I was at one end of a lane. My brother was at the other end, in an armchair, singing sentimental songs. I walked up the lane but when he saw me, he suddenly got up and drove away on a scooter, leaving me alone. It was night-time and I was afraid. As I was walking on the lonely road, four or five men suddenly began to chase me. I was very scared, ran as fast as I could, managed to reach a safe place and shut the doors before they could catch me.

[16/f]

Disease

■ I am shocked to discover, while bathing, that my entire leg is covered with small, round, black eruptions crowded together (like bees on a honey comb). I am "dead scared" and call out to my husband. When he rubs my

foot, the eruptions on that part just vanish.

[A3/m]

■ I lift up my sleeve to discover that I have some horrible skin disease on my left arm. There are many pink, small and softish appearing eruptions on my forearm. I do not touch them. I feel disgusted with myself, and feel as if this arm is not a part of me. I hold the arm away from my body and go to see a doctor. While she is examining me, I am shocked to see more such papular eruptions right upto the axilla, some of them large and "flowering". One of the eruptions is large, fleshy, pedunculated and dimpled in the centre; it is of a yellow colour like picric acid kept in a glass bottle. The doctor informs me that my disease is somewhat incurable. I feel very frustrated. I visit another doctor who tells me that gradually the disease will disappear by excising the growths. I am terrified with the thought of the pain.

I had the feeling throughout the dream as if I had been scratching my arm.

[A 40/f]

■ Having a discussion with an asthmatic woman, and asking her how she feels during the attacks. I tell her that I used to get irritable.

[A 15/f]

■ I do something to one of the many children who are on a lawn, and the child begins to pursue me down a slope and throw things on me. Then he opens a kitchen store from which he removes hot metal objects, and tries to throw them upon me. I am suddenly naked and scared of being burnt. I run until I come to a precipice, and try to climb down.

Then I am suddenly on a kind of terrace paved with marble stones. In front of me there is a river in which there are three suitcases swimming. Two men emerge on the surface, open one of the suitcases, get into it and shut it. I wonder how these big men can fit into so small a suitcase, but I see the same thing being repeated with the second suitcase.

Then I see a man emerge from a stone house. He has an eczema on his right cheek, which is oozing a sticky, red fluid. I begin to follow a woman who wants to guide me to another place. The man holds me back and tells me that he will not let me go until I have kissed him on his right cheek. I am disgusted but I obey as I want to escape from him. But now he is less inclined to let me go, even though the woman says a magic formula. I feel he is holding me with a metal and can feel a dull pain on the right side of the nape and inner angle of the right scapula. I wake from the dream on purpose disgusted, and still able to feel the pain. I am afraid to fall asleep again with the fear that he will catch me once again.

[17'/f]

▪ I am given a packet of X-Rays, which show that I have cavitatory tuberculosis. I was frightened. Felt as if I was groping in the dark, did not trust the data.

[29/m]

Miscellaneous

▪ I was squeezing past flowering bushes when walking along a narrow garden path. The bushes were linked together by webs. I managed to get past the bushes by jumping over, or squeezing, or brushing past them, but having done that I realized that there was no road on the other side as I had expected. I had to turn back and found that the bushes were now bigger and I would have to jump over these obstacles to get back.

Suddenly, two of my teachers appeared and asked me to identify the flowers on the bushes. With some difficulty I managed to identify them as Digitalis – the fox glove. My teachers were unhappy about the amount of time I took over the answer. I felt ashamed when they told me about how much trouble they went through to teach students and yet we hardly knew anything. I felt guilty, as if I had been caught when trying to escape.

[A18/m]

▪ Playing a game similar to soccer. I was on the attacking side and my captain wanted me to hit the ball fast and perfectly, to win the game.

[A 34/f]

▪ My mother is scolding me for being rude and is asking me to change my behaviour. I am both hurt and astonished as to how she could tell me this.

[18'/f]

▪ I am in the kitchen one morning, wearing only stretch pants. I know that soon the cook and my uncle will come and I should rush back to my room and cover myself. I pull the stretch pants over my torso and run to my bedroom.

[B 4/f]

▪ I give my son a pair of half-trousers. He wears them with his shirt tucked in. The trousers are from his chest right down to his knees, and right above the waist they are frilled like women's clothes. My son doesn't like his attire. He asks me what kind of clothes I am giving him. I tell him that a famous homoeopath has stitched them and so he should wear them. I convince him to wear them, maybe as we convince patients.

Suddenly I see masons working at some building work. One of them tells the others that my son is a foreigner because of his attire. It seemed to be only a comment, rather than a mockery, but my son pulls his shirt out of the trousers so that it hangs down to his knees, over the trousers.

[20/m]

▪ I have married my childhood sweetheart, and am travelling with her to a distant place because my parents have driven me out of the house.

[A'12/m]

▪ Parents drive me out of the house because I did not clear my exams.

[A'12/m]

▪ My father and brother were quarrelling because of my brother's poor exam scores. My father asks my brother to leave the house and my brother is ready to go. I tell my father that henceforth I will help my brother with his studies so that he scores well. But neither of them listen to me. I feel sorry that I am unable to do anything.

[D1/m]

• We were all youngsters in the pre-independance period. We went to a large urinal that was dirty, unwashed. I could not urinate because of the dirt.

Then I went to another building where there was a two-way radio. I asked my friend whether I could hear radio programmes on it. He said I could try.

Then we started to walk towards the urinal. As we approached the gate, we saw that the building had been attacked by British soldiers, so that they could nab freedom fighters.

Then the scene shifted to a library during the period of British rule. I saw my friend there. I asked him how come he was free. He answered that he simply became a member of the British Library.

[31/m]

• Some persons had to prepare a report about a place, the sands of which had never been tread upon. It was a large, sandy area and the horses could walk it with ease. The report that they prepared was good.

[A 26/m]

• Going on an adventure in a jungle, full of excitement.

[A 31/m]

• I am in my house. There are two paths that lead to it, one of which is supposed to be haunted by a ghost or spirit. The building next to my house is also haunted. Whenever I come home, someone along that haunted path calls me to the haunted house; it is irresistible. I ask my family members to help me face the ghost, but no one except my brother agrees to come with me to the haunted house and unravel its mystery. I am not in the least afraid.

[D 13/f]

• Oriental children with their heads shaved, and dressed up like monks are inside a house. An Oriental woman is holding them captive, and is forcing them to do something. The house has two doors. The frontdoor is guarded by armed men. One of the boys manages to evade the woman and escape through the back door. He is running downhill, when he is joined by a young woman in Oriental garb, who encourages him to run fast. They continue to run till they come to a flight of steps which they climb. At the top of the stairs, there is a cupboard next to a house. The woman opens the door of the cupboard and there are two short, weird looking, divine people inside. The woman places the boy in the midst of these two people or Gods, and gives him some advice regarding his mother. Then she closes the door.

I get the idea that this small boy will become a great monk.

[25/m]

• Dreams of laboured efforts, of fatigue.

[A1/m]

• Wanting to teach students better, so that something definite can be achieved and Homoeopathy evolves.

[B 2/m]

• Trying to swim in a vast ocean. My younger sisters are swimming towards the horizon and my friend encourages me to try and catch up with them. I am trying, but am being thrown out and away although my sisters are succeeding.

• Someone measuring land using measuring tape.

[A6/m]

• Money bag.

[A 28/f]

▪ We have moved into a large house which resembles a hotel. It has large rooms, a high ceiling, big pieces of furniture, and tall curtains. The distance between the front door and the hall is a hundred feet. I reproach myself on being foolish to buy a place that is going to be difficult to maintain.

[A 32/f]

▪ My neighbour who lives abroad has bought a new car – a red Contessa. The car is gift-wrapped in cardboard and a red ribbon tied into a bow. Her family members and other neighbours have surrounded the car, and I am watching from above.

[C3/f]

▪ I am emptying the contents of my brother's suitcase and find six toothbrushes amongst them. I feel I will dispose my old toothbrush and use a new one henceforth. I also find a wooden spoon wrapped in a transparent plastic bag, and call out to my mother telling her that my brother has bought it for her. But when I pick it up to my surprise I find it broken and wonder how my brother could have bought a broken spoon.

[C3/f]

▪ I was in a big hall, shopping with my mother, when I discovered a piano. I was happy and started to play a Chopin waltz which I knew by heart, but after three or four measures I could not remember how to play it anymore. I tried to start again but after three or four attempts I gave up, saddened and disappointed.

Afterwards a man bought another old piano and started to take it apart. My friend appeared and told me that both pianos belonged to her, and that she wanted to make one good piano out of the best pieces of the two older ones. I thought it was a good idea, but felt sadness and envy that she had two pianos, while I had none.

[17'/f]

▪ My husband and I were visiting the house of a friend in an Indian town. There we saw a number of people touching the feet of an elderly man. We thought it was some celebration, but to my surprise I was informed that this was a large joint family comprising of fifty persons and this was their daily ritual. I wondered how such a large family adjusted amongst each other, the size of their kitchen, the number of telephones they possessed, etc.

[A 32/f]

▪ I am bowing down to my mother-in law with a feeling of tremendous respect for her from within. Then I bow down to my father and feel a lot of reverance, as if these are very revered people (to me), I value them and they are so nice and good.

[19'/m]

▪ I was walking down a crowded street on a rainy day. A middle-aged man came near me and taking advantage of the crowd, tried to misbehave with me. I looked at him angrily and in disgust, but he smiled back shamelessly. I got very angry, and began to hit him with my umbrella. When he tried to run, I ran after him and continued to hit him, till finally someone had to stop me. I told people around that such persons take advantage if girls keep quiet and that they should not be allowed to get away and should be taught a lesson.

[D13/f]

▪ A revered professor was trying to make sexual advances at my niece. We were in the same van, like cousins, and he was trying to lift her skirt up and trying to touch her breasts. I was watching from far and I wondered why such a revered person was doing this, and why she was allowing it to happen to her.

[19'/m]

▪ I was attending a seminar with my friends. Just before it started, my friend who was seated next to me left his chair and went to speak with another participant. A teacher for whom I have no respect occupied my friend's seat. I was surprised, unpleasantly, and politely informed him that someone else had been sitting in that seat. But my friend said that it was okay with him, and sat down elsewhere. I was very uncomfortable to be sitting next to this professor, and felt that I would be forced to interact with him. So I tried to trick him to go away by reminding him that he was a guest invitee and that he should be sitting in the front rows. I went up to the organizers and asked that he be made to sit up front, but they said it was okay if he sat behind. I realized that my trick had failed.

[B 1/m]

* Going from place to place in a deserted, big building like a palace. I saw the rooms, mostly from a height with fascination on the one hand and sorrow on the other.

[A1/m]

▪ Of being at the ruins of an old fort, a historical place in Mahabaleshwar, where a dynamite was being exploded to unearth something. Patches of the roof of a building in the same premises began to fall as a result of the explosion; they were like segments of a jig-saw puzzle and had prints of tiger painting on them. While I was trying to save myself from being hit by those pieces, I was at the same time trying to collect them.

[A9/m]

▪ Bringing about peace between colleagues of my department amongst whom there were differences of opinion.

[A 11/m]

▪ Raping a junior colleague because she had teased me.

[A' 12/m]

▪ Threatening my professor that I would kill him if he failed me.

[A' 12/m]

▪ Usual dreams of losing confidence in myself and realizing the superiority of the other person when a challenge was thrown to me, were ameliorated. Had an unusually calm sleep.

[A 17/m]

▪ I was amongst a large number of people standing together in the stock market. Someone asked me to be the president of an institution. I replied that I wasn't interested, and that being a chairman or president was nothing new to me since I had always functioned in that way.

[A 26/m]

▪ An assembly of people were appreciating one man for his honesty and integrity.

[A 26/m]

▪ A group of people have come under the power of a tyrant like Hitler. He has passed a decree that all people will be killed after they have cleansed themselves by passing a stool either naturally or with the help of an enema or purgative. I am the last one in a queue of people and so I escape, because the time is up and the killer squad has already packed up and left the scene.

[A 32/f]

▪ I am amongst a group which is partaking in an experiment to determine the effect of different items of food, especially, vegetables, on the mental characteristics of patient. A person is given only tomatoes, and his behaviour observed, and so on.

[A 32/f]

▪ I wanted to go out with my sister-in-law in the morning. She was waiting for me to get dressed, but something went wrong for which my father scolded me and my mother gave me some domestic work to do, and so I could not go out. Under my mother's instructions, I was about to put turmeric powder[1] into a bottle, when I noticed it was slightly wet. I kept the bottle in the sunlight to dry when I noticed a very tiny man, some four to five inches tall, come out of the bottle. He started to run away when I quickly caught him by the shirt and pulled him back, telling him that he thought too much of himself and

---

1   Spice used in Indian cooking.

that I wouldn't let him escape. I forcibly put him back into the bottle, happy and excited, while the others around me laughed at his defeat.

[D 13/f]

▪ All my hair has suddenly gone grey. I look in the mirror with surprise and realize that I need to dye it.

[B 4/f]

▪ I go to a woman's house to buy a dupatta [1]. Half the people in her house belong to her family, while the other half belong to another family. The woman tells me that she does not have the dupattas presently as they are in someone else's house.

Then my father comes and invites them for tea, which the man in the house politely refuses. As my father leaves, the man addresses him by another name and I correct him. We have casual conversation for a while and then as I get up to leave, the woman hands me a packet which is supposed to be a tablet she had borrowed from my mother. I open the packet to find plenty of sewing needles, and jokingly ask her if she intended to poke needles in our family matter.

[C 3/f]

▪ My brother-in-law told me that both his phones were out of order, and although he had personally made complaints to the officers in charge it was of no use.

[A 32/f]

▪ There was a fire in my house in which an important document was partially burnt.

[A 32/f]

▪ I am getting late to attend a seminar because I take long to get dressed, and then my brother who is to reach me is performing a religious ritual. He says he will reach me after fifteen minutes and I tell him that it will

---

1   Piece of cloth similar to a scarf, draped over the shoulders and covering the torso, and sometimes even the head; an essential part of the Indian's woman attire.

be too late.

[A 32/f]

▪ I wake up fifteen minutes after the time that my examination had been scheduled. I am very anxious that I won't be able to finish the exam. I ask my husband how he allowed me to oversleep. I am very rushed, am not ready with my clothes. I ask one of my servants to get me a handkerchief, and another to get me a taxi.

[A 32/f]

▪ Writing down a case that two of my professors are taking.

[A 35/f]

▪ Events of the day.

[C 4/m]

▪ Riding my old bicycle.

[C 4/m]

▪ Recall the rubric, "Fear of being injured", while a teacher is teaching on a stage with three or four students around him.

[D 2/m]

▪ Of being near a truck with a pail of dirty water.

[D 8/m]

▪ Workers from a coal mine are bathing in separate wooden cubicles. I feel that no matter how much they try to clean themselves, they will remain black.

[25/m]

▪ A graveyard where a funeral is being held, and a party going on just beside it.

[26/m]

▪ My sister wanted my hair clip. It sat crooked in her hair, while it sat straight in mine.

[D9/f]

▪ I had gone to some office, in disguise. I wanted to search for some proof so that I could take revenge against somebody. Suddenly I realized that someone had recognized me and I start to run until finally I reached a safe place.

[D 10/f]

- I am watching TV. The picture is of an empty playground which has been shot from a height. Suddenly a leather ball appears on the ground and someone tells me that there is a game going on at some distance from the ground during which a player has hit the ball out of their field and scored six runs.

[D 12/m]

- I am working in an allopathic hospital, and a person I know has been admitted as a patient. One of my neighbours is doing the rounds. She is a not a medical person but she makes a scene that I do not know any medicine, and advises me to start the patient on a diuretic drip.

[D 12/m]

- Fighting for my rights, for justice. Someone is telling me that I deserve it and that I should get it.

[D 13/f]

- Sitting at the window of a bus while travelling. Suddenly, I saw a big blue waterfall.

[D4/f]

- Running about in the college hostel and canteen.

[E 1/f]

- A pond of water into which a ball-like object which resembled in the earth, splashed in.

[16/f]

- A merry-go-round with many grown up people sitting or standing on it. To get it going faster, one had to turn it while running around it, and then jump onto the platform. I did the same although the platform was already crowded, and I was turning clockwise for a long time.

[17'/f]

PHYSICAL SYMPTOMS

Generalities

- Desire to eat things rich in cream and milk on waking from sleep during the night.

[A26]

- Very strong craving for eggs.

[20/m]

- Dullness, physical, as well as mental.

[A1/m]

- Sensitivity to least touch.

[D1/m]

- Pains all over the body at night.

[I/m]

- Fatigue; felt "sapped" out of energy.

[I/m]

- Sleep ameliorates.

[A4/f]

- Energetic despite sleeplessness.

[A5/m]

- Weak, totally exhausted feeling.

[C2/f]

- Energetic, despite lack of sleep. Especially energetic after 11.00 a.m.

[A10/m

- Disinclination for exertion.

[A11/m]

- Fatigue, as if I had done some physical work.

[D3/f]

- Tiredness.

[D15/f]

- Feverish feeling with desire to lie down.

[A3/*]

- Energetic.
[A37/f]

- Extraordinary weakness in the evening.
[7/m]

- Hot feeling.
[16/f]

- Warm wave travelling through the right arm, and then through the left arm.
[A'35/f]

- Activity mental and physical, increased, especially in the evening without any feeling of exhaustion.
[A'35/f]

Physical particulars

Vertigo

- Vertigo, in the morning, on rising. Unable to stand, to walk straight.
[A4/f]

- Vertigo, ameliorated lying supine. Aggravated lying on sides. Vertigo as if the bed was swaying, and I would fall off the bed.
[D12/m]

- Mild giddiness, imbalance.
[7/m]

Head

- Dull headache from occiput to parietal region.
[D1/m]

- Severe aching in frontal skull bones, on waking.
[E3/f]

- Heaviness in the head.
[A6/m]

- Empty feeling in the head, on waking in the morning.
[A8/m]

- Right temporal headache.
[A8/m]

- Pain in frontal sinuses.
[C2/f]

- Frontal headache.
[C3/f]

- Left-sided, throbbing pain in morning. Spread up to occiput in afternoon. Settled in vertex and frontal regional in the evening. Aggravated from movements, walking, music, noise, fanning. Ameliorated from pressure.
[C4/m]

- Eruptions forehead, on the back of the head, four to five, sensitive to touch.
[A 11/m]

- Heaviness in the head, especially frontal, as from a weight.
[A'12/m]

- Pain in forehead and supra-orbital regions.
[A 15/f]

- Heaviness in the head.
[A 15/f]

- Aching in occiput and vertex. Worse travelling in bus.
[A 15/f]

- Dull headache since morning, throughout the day. Ameliorated from rest, closing the eyes, evening.
[B3/f]

- Dull, frontal headache.
[B5/m]

- Feeling of constriction in the forehead and temples.
[A9/m]

- Shooting pain in right temple, lasting one or two seconds, coming and going in paroxysms. Better from holding the hand against the head.
[16/f]

- Feeling of tension in the head.
  [7/m]
- Dull aching pain, frontal.
  [D9/f]
- Severe throbbing pain in the right temple. Worse at 4 p.m., noise, light, pressure. Headache accompanied by nausea.
  [A 19/f]
- Headache at 10.30 a.m.; heavy, dull feeling in the head lasting for an hour.
  [D 13/f]
- Intense headache in the vertex, over the right eye, at 11 a.m. Heavy, dull feeling, throbbing, especially on the right side of the head. Better from walking. Worse from reading, sitting quiet, pressure. Headache accompanied by giddiness. The headache was so severe that I couldn't concentrate on anything. Subdued after sleep, but returned on attempting to read.
  [D 13/f]
- Dull pain in vertex and forehead on waking in the morning. Better as the day passed, from pressure, hot bath and rapid motion.
  [A23/f]
- Head pain, left side, radiating from occiput to vertex; throbbing, stitching. Comes suddenly, last a few seconds, disappears suddenly. Pain ameliorated from rapid motion.
  [A23/f]
- Severe pain in forehead and vertex, constant. Ameliorated by pressure, hot water bath, rapid motion.
  [A23/f]
- Pimples – left side of forehead.
  [A25/f]
- Old symptom of heaviness in the head on ascending reappeared.
  [A28/f]
- Occipital headache in the morning.
  [A36/f]
- Heaviness in the head, better in the afternoon.
  [A36/f]
- Dull, frontal pain in the afternoon.
  [A 35/f]

Eye / Vision

- Heaviness and burning in the eyes.
  [E1/f]
- Small, painful swelling on the inner side of right upper eyelid.
  [E1/f]
- Desire to close the eyes.
  [E1/f]
- Severe aching in eyelids, on waking.
  [E2/f]
- Heaviness of eyelids; unable to open the eyes.
  [E2/f]
- Discomfort, swelling right eye. Sensitivity of skin and bone in one spot around the socket.
  [A 11/m]
- Burning sensation in the right eye.
  [A 11/m]
- Lower lid of left eye seemed lax, so that it seemed that eye movements were uncoordinated.
  [A22/m]
- Heaviness of eyes, with heaviness of the head.
  [A 36/f]

Ears and hearing

- Partial blocking of both ears since rising from bed, remaining the whole day.
  [A4/f]
- Severe shooting pain in right ear which had been deaf since the last three years.
  [A9/m]
- Pulling pain in the right ear.
  [B3/f]

Nose and smell

- "Blockage" of right nostril, while

rising.

[D1/m]

- Frequent sneezing throughout the day. Worse in cold air, draught.

[D1/f]

- Red discolouration at the tip of the nose.

[A5/m]

- Sneezing.

[C2/f]

- Watery coryza.

[C2/f]

- Thick, white, sticky coryza.

[C2/f]

- Blocked nose.

[C2/f]

- Itching in the right nostril.

[A27/f]

- Continuous sneezing in the morning.

[A27/f]

- Previous symptom of thick, yellow coryza was very much ameliorated.

[A30/m]

- Pressure in left nostril, lasting for one minute.

[A'35/f]

- Severe bouts of sneezing in the morning, and before going to bed.

[A 35/f]

- Sneezing attacks without coryza.

[D12/m]

- Catarrh.

[19'/m]

Face

- Perspiration at the angles of the mouth.

[D1/m]

- Vascular eruption over left cheek – non-itching.

[A5/m]

- A big, painful boil between the eyebrows.

[A9/m]

- Mild itching on right cheek, left nasal fold, lasting twelve hours.

[A 24/f]

Mouth and taste

- Aphtous ulcer on the inside of the upper lip with a yellow point, with redness of the surrounding area. Very painful to touch, stitching type of pain.

[C1/m]

- Burning upper palate.

[D1/m]

- Excessive bleeding from gums.

[A9/m]

- Dryness of mouth.

[A'2/f]

- Coated tongue.

[A'12/m]

- Foul breath.

[A'12/m]

- Profuse foul smelling salivation on waking in morning.

[B3/f]

- Salty tasting sputum.

[A18/m]

Throat

- Burning in throat.

[D1/m]

- Constrictive feeling in the throat.

[E1/f]

- Ticking sensation in throat, which excites cough.

[E1/f]

- Pricking sensation in the right side of the throat, worse at night.

[E 4/f]

- Burning, itching, irritation, redness in throat. Worse from swallowing. Better from hot drinks.

[C2/f]

- Post nasal discharge.

[C2/f]

- Pain in throat, radiating to the ears.
  [C2/f]
- Congestion.
  [A13/f]
- Irritation in the throat at night.
  [E1/f]
- Dryness in throat pit, at night.
  [A31/m]
- Soreness in the throat, with cough.
  [B4/m]
- Pain.
  [q0'/m

External throat

- Itching of the right side of neck, posteriorly.
  [A14/m]
- Small, red, painful eruptions on neck.
  [D7/f]
- Mild itching on the front of neck, lasting for half an hour.
  [D7/f]
- Neck pain as if strained, from lying on side; was compelled to lie on the back.
  [A 34/f]

Stomach

- Increased appetite.
  [D1/m]
- Nausea.
  [D1/m]
- Thirst for large quantities, infrequently.
  [D1/m]
- Burning in the stomach.
  [D1/m]
- Nausea.
  [A4/f]
- Decreased appetite.
  [A4/f]
- Nausea at the sight of food.
  [E3/f]

- Vomiting, yellow, of undigested food at 2.30 a.m., on waking from a dream of strangulation.
  [C3/f]
- Empty sensation in the stomach from tea (which he desired).
  [20/m]
- Appetite reduced, with heaviness in the stomach.
  [A10/m]
- Nausea, with headache.
  [A19/f]
- Increased appetite.
  [D 15/f]
- Thirst increased, for cold water.
  [D 27/]
- Thirst at night; had to wake from sleep.
  [A 31/m]
- Decreased appetite.
  [A8/m]

Abdomen

- Severe cutting pain in the abdomen, from right to left. Ameliorated from pressure.
  [D1/m]
- Flatulent distention of the abdomen.
  [E1/f]
- Red, itching macular eruptions.
  [A5/m]
- Sudden, sharp pain in the right hypogastric region, from laughing or from jar.
  [E3/f]
- Extreme uneasiness in abdomen, gaseous distension; abdomen felt tense in the evening.
  [E3/f]
- Sensation as if intestines were being pulled from inside.
  [E3/f]
- Tenesmus at 3.00 a.m.; had to rush for stool.
  [E2/f]

- Heaviness.
[A10/m]

- Pain in inguinal and umbilical regions.
[D7/f]

- Uneasiness in the abdomen, along with distention.
[A19/f]

- Pain in the morning, before stool.
[A37/f]

- Old symptom of itching in the groins was very much aggravated and violent.
[A26/m]

- Constricting sensation in left abdomen, near umbilical region, along with dull aching pain.
[A35'/f]

- Cramping pain.

Rectum and stool

- Mild diarrhoea.
[25/m]

- Hard stool, difficult to pass.
[D1/m]

- Irregular stool, every alternate day.
[D1/m]

- Stools: loose, watery, yellow, dark, lumpy.
[E2/f]

- Tears while passing stool.
[E2/f]

- Stool offensive, accompanied by flatus.
[A5/m]

- Initial part of stool required straining.
[A9/m]

- Greenish coloured stools.
[C3/f]

- Mucus in stools. Stools frequent, required straining.
[C4/m]

- Constipation, severe.
[A112/m]

- Sudden, irresistible urge to pass stool in the evening.
[D12/m]

- Forcible diarrhoea with immense burning in the rectum; thought I might collapse.
[D2/m]

- Severe diarrhoea in the morning.
[A19/f]

- Sudden, painless urging for stool, while eating groundnuts.
[20/m]

- Ineffectual urging for stool.
[25/m]

Bladder and urination

- Frequency of urination.
[A10/m]

Cough

- Cough at night; forceful, in bouts.
[E4/f]

- Dry cough.
[A'12/m]

- Severe, dry cough, lasting for half an hour after dose.
[A30/m]

- Cough in the morning.
[A36/f]

Expectoration

- Morning expectoration thick, yellow, like a band or thread.
[D1/m]

- Salty expectoration.
[A 18/m]

Chest

- Itching eruptions in the right axilla.
[E1/f]

- Retrosternal dull ache, three episodes in a day, each lasting ten minutes.
[E3/f]

- Excessive, terrible pain in the heart, in the region of the left ventricle; felt if I could remove the heart and keep it aside, I would feel better. Ameliorated between 4.00 p.m. and 6 p.m.

[C3/f]

- Palpitations on waking in the morning.
[B3/f]

- Layer of white material on the areola of both breasts, as if some milk had oozed out and dried up.

[D 12/m]

- Pain, left side of chest.
[A 27/f]

- Sensation of right sticking in between the ribs left in the region of the heart lasting one minute. Worse lying down. Desire to press the ribs.

[A'35/f]

- Left-sided chest pain, from frequent sneezing.

[D1/m]

Back
- Dull pain in back. Ameliorated from stretching the shoulder forward. Worse from continuous sitting.

[D1/m]

- Itching on back, on going to sleep.
[A34/f]

- Low backache.

[A25/f]

Extremities
- Pain in the legs, ameliorated from motion, worse during the night.

[1/m]

- Itching eruptions, right forearm.
[E1/f]

- Weakness, severe pain in the lower extremities. Worse sitting, walking.
[A6/m]

- Pain in the hip joints.
[A6/m]

- Tiredness, cramps in the lower extremities.

[A6/m]

- Small, pimple-like eruptions in both cubital fossae.

[E4/f]

- Dry, eczematous, itching eruptions on both hands.

[D3/m]

- Cramps, upper and lower extremities.
[A8/m]

- Severe pain in the left popliteal fossa. Aggravated from walking, sleeping. Better from sitting.

[A 12/m]

- Numbness: index and middle finger of right hand, at 4.45 a.m.

[A14/m]

- Itching, left knee at 6 a.m.
[A14/m]

- Small, red, painful eruptions on forearm.
[D7/f]

- Heaviness of feet, sense of inability to lift them.

[D7/f]

- Old symptom of itching in dorsum of foot reappeared.

[A28/f]

- Red, itching, round eruptions on foot.
[A29/f]

- Heat of palms.

[A'35/f]

- Severe pain in the hand from slight touch, oversensitive.

[D1/m]

- Pain in the right lower extremity.
[25/m]

Sleep
- Disturbed sleep; uneasy and restless all night, was tossing and turning.

[1/m]

- Sleeplessness.

[A5/m]

- Sleep disturbed.

[A6/m]

- Drowsiness, sleepiness throughout the day, with inability to concentrate.

[D4/f]

- Sleep unrefreshed.

[D4/f]

- Disturbed sleep, waking up anxious, waking difficult.

[C3]

- Disturbed sleep.

[A10/m]

- Sleepless till 1.30 a.m.

[A10/m]

- Sleepiness on attempting to read.

[A 12/m]

- Drowsy (through someone commented I look fresh).

[D9/f]

- Unusually very calm sleep.

[A17/m]

- Disturbed at 3.00 a.m.

[A 24/f]

- Waking frequently.

[A24/f]

- Drowsiness.

[D5/m]

- Sleepless till 1.30 - 2.00 a.m.

[A25/f]

- Sleepy in the evening.

[D30/*]

- Sleeplessness due to activity of the mind.

[A27/f]

- Sleepiness throughout the day and night.

[A29/f]

- Late to fall asleep.

[A39/f]

- Waking frequently.

[A39/f]

- Increased sleep, especially mornings and evenings.

[D14/*]

Fever

- Fever with chills at 4 a.m.

[A3/*]

- Fever with malaise, and great weakness.

[19'/m]

Skin

- Itching in very small spot, especially on the right side of the body.

[A'35/f]

RUBRICS

Mind

Single symptoms

— Antagonism with herself, constant, sympathetic and helpful, whether she should be, or selfish and self-centred.

— Antagonism with herself, individuality versus group, conformity, about.

— Company, desire for, attract others towards himself, wanted to.

— Company, desire for, group, old, wants to belong to, again.

— Confidence, want of self, daytime.

— Confidence, want of self, evening ameliorates.

— Delusion, friends, he had done a lot for his, and got nothing in return.

— *Delusion, friends, unwanted by.*

— Delusion, self-centred, all others were.

— Delusion, worthless, that he was.

— Dreams, animals, cat, big, white.

— Dreams, animals, huge.

— Dreams, animals, lion.

— Dreams, animals, panther.

— Dreams, animals, python, encircled the abdomen of her pregnant friend.

— Dreams, animals, snakes, golden.

— Dreams, animals, snakes, tiny.

— Dreams, animals, snakes, surrounded by.

— Dreams, animals, snakes, of killing.

— Dreams, animals, snakes, escape him.

— Dreams, animals, snakes, converted into liquid.

— Dreams, assisting a sick stranger.

— Dreams, bicycle riding, his old.

— Dreams, bluish discharge from nostril.

— Dreams, body, body parts, hair, greying of.

— Dreams, body, body parts, leg, covered with eruptions.

— Dreams, bridge, of crossing, over flooded river.

— Dreams, buildings, palatial, of wandering in.

— Dreams, childbirth, premature.

— Dreams, childbirth, distressing.

— Dreams, children, babies, healthy though premature.

— Dreams, children, held captive.

— Dreams, cliff, he is at the edge of a.

— Dreams, clothes, convincing his son to wear unusual clothes.

— Dreams, consoling his teacher.

— Dreams, classroom, being turned out of.

— **Dreams, cousins**

— Dreams, cousin, emaciated.

— Dreams, cousin, fearful, of reassuring.

— Dreams, cousin, handicapped, she was helping.

— Dreams, cousin, she is scolding.

— Dreams, cousin, teaching, younger cousins.

— Dreams, criminal, escaping, even though roped in tightly.

— Dreams, danger, family, to his.

— Dreams, death, fear of, replaced by an acceptance.

— *Dreams, deserted, of being.*

— Dreams, disaster, averted, being.

— Dreams, disease, incurable, of having.

— Dreams, disease, cousin.

— Dreams, disgusted with herself, of being.

— Dreams, efforts to evolve his subject.

— Dreams, escaping from captivity to become a great monk.

— Dreams, experiments with human beings.

— Dreams, faces, horrible.

— Dreams, family, large.

— Dreams, families, two different, living in the same house.

— Dreams, fights, fighting a man who attacked his group.

— Dreams, fights, fighting, rights, for.

— Dreams, floods, streets flooded.

— Dreams, forest, of roaming in a.

— *Dreams, forsaken, of being.*

— *Dreams, friends, alone, left, by.*

— Dreams, friends, assisting a sick friend.

— Dreams, friends, company of, being in.

— *Dreams, friends, of helping his.*

— Dreams, friends, punished by.

— Dreams, fun, by hurting others.

— Dreams, funerals and parties.

— Dreams, girl forsaken by her boyfriend.

— Dreams, game, team captain, wants him to win.

— Dreams, guilt, of not feeling.

— Dreams, held back by a disgusting man.

— Dreams, helped, being, strangers, by.

— Dreams, helpful, being, rather than think of himself which he later regretted.

— Dreams, high places, ledge, hanging from.

— Dreams, home, turned out of.

— Dreams, journeys, road, through deserted.

— Dreams, journeys, road, with ups and downs.

— Dreams, journeys, train derailing.

— Dreams, journeys, friends, with.

— *Dreams, journeys, trains.*

— Dreams, killed, that everyone should be, decree had been passed.

— Dreams, labour, of conducting.

— Dreams. land being measured.

— Dreams, lonely, of feeling.

— Dreams, man, tiny, trapped in a bottle.

— Dreams, man, striking, for having misbehaved with her.

— Dreams, men, big, small suitcases, in.

— Dreams, mother, asking for milk.

— Dreams, mountain, snow-covered.

— Dreams, murder, cousin, being murdered.

— Dreams, nakedness, she must cover herself.

— Dreams, nakedness, being naked when alone.

— Dreams, nakedness, she and her friends were naked, surprised that she felt no embarrassment.

— Dreams, needle, accidently, he swallowed.

— Dreams, obstacles, path, in his.

— Dreams, peace, of making, between quarrelling friends.

— Dreams, people, assembly of, appreciating the honesty and integrity of a prominent person.

— Dreams, pianos, her friend had two, while she had none.

— Dreams, politely trying to get an undesirable person to move away.

— Dreams, processions, giant.

— Dreams, pursued, elephant, by.

— Dreams, pursued, teased, and, men, by.

— Dreams, quarrels, friend, with.

— Dreams, relatives, visiting.

— Dreams, reporting an untread place.

— Dreams, reprimanded, friend, by.

— Dreams, reprimanded, mother, by, rude behaviour, for.

— Dreams, reprimanded, teacher, by.

— Dreams, rescued, brother, by.

— Dreams, religion, disapproval at persons from different religions sitting together.

— Dreams, revered person being sexually abusive.

— Dreams, reverance to elders.

— Dreams, riots, communal (inter-religious).

— Dreams, ritually showing respect to an elder family member.

— Dreams, road, curved.

— Dreams, ruins, historical places, of.

— Dreams, sand castles, of building.

— Dreams, saved by person of rival community.

— Dreams, saints, different religions from, coming together.

— Dreams, shameless, of being.

— Dreams, soiling clothes.

— Dreams, speeding, of.

— Dreams, sympathizing with forsaken friend.

— Dreams, threats, threatening to kill his teacher.

— Dreams, tyrant, of being under the power of a.

— Dreams, umbilical cord, she did not sever.

— Dreams, unsuccessful efforts, swim, to.

— Dreams, visit, social.

— Dreams, water, dirty.

— Dreams, water, sea, bathing in.

— Dreams, wedding, cousin, of.

— Dreams, weeping from reprimands.

— Dreams, woman, guiding her.

— Dreams, work, improving, at.

— Dullness, sluggishness, difficulty in thinking, afternoon.

— Hurry, haste, driving, while, overtake all others, with a desire to.

— Indolence, aversion to work, alternating with industriousness.

— Impulse, burn matchsticks, to.

— Impulse morbid, harm loved ones to, even though the very thought caused him to shudder.

— Impulse, morbid, throttle, a teacher, to, sudden.

— Injures himself.

— Irritability, mother, to her.

— Killed, she would rather be than left alone.

— Lamenting, futility of human relationships, about.

— Reverence, teacher, towards his.

— Thoughts, persistent, work, of improving, at, alternating with thoughts of leisure.

— Weary of life, existence seems painful.

— Weeping, tearful mood, afternoon, 5.00 p.m.

— Weeping, tearful mood, kindness of others, when thinking of.

— Will, contradiction, work and rest, about.

— Wills two, feels as if he had two wills, one urging him to be God fearing and religious, while the other prompts him to be unreligious and sinful.

Common symptoms
- Anger, alternating with quick repentance.
- Anger, contradiction from.
- Anger, will, if things do not go after his.
- Answers, monosyllabic.
- *Antagonism with herself.*
- Anxiety, conscience, of.
- Anxiety, trifles, from.
- Capriciousness.
- Company, aversion to, desire for solitude.
- Company, desire for.
- Concentration, difficult.
- Confidence, increased.
- Confidence, self, in.
- Confusion of mind.
- Conscientious, trifles, about.
- Contradiction, intolerant of.
- Conversation, ameliorates.
- Death, desires.
- Death, thoughts of.
- *Delusion, alone always.*
- Delusion, alone in the world.
- Delusion, friendless, that he is.
- *Delusion, neglected, she is.*
- Delusion, wrong, he has done.
- Despair, life, of.
- Dictatorial.
- Dreams, accusations, crime, wrongful, of.
- Dreams, adventurous.
- Dreams, animals.
- Dreams, animals, fishes.
- Dreams, animals, rats.
- *Dreams, animals, snakes.*
- Dreams, animals, wild.
- Dreams, anxious.
- Dreams, astray, of going.
- Dreams, blood.
- Dreams, body, body parts, arm covered with blisters.
- Dreams, cars, automobiles, of.
- Dreams, childbirth, of.
- Dreams, children, babies, of.
- Dreams, danger, death, of.
- Dreams, dead relatives.
- Dreams, death, friend, of a.
- Dreams, disease, loathsome.
- Dreams, disease, sick people.
- Dreams, disease, sick people, mother, his.
- Dreams, disgusting.
- Dreams, eating.
- Dreams, exertion.
- Dreams, examinations.
- Dreams, falling, danger, of.
- Dreams, fights.
- Dreams, fire.
- Dreams, fleeing
- Dreams, flood.
- Dreams, flying.
- Dreams, frightful.
- Dreams, gardens.
- Dreams, hiding from danger.
- Dreams, high places.
- **Dreams, journeys**.
- Dreams, laughing.
- Dreams, money.
- Dreams, murder.
- Dreams, parties, of, pleasure.
- Dreams, picnics.
- Dreams, poisoned, of being.
- Dreams, praying.
- Dreams, pursued.

— Dreams, quarrels.

— Dreams, rape, that he has committed.

— Dreams, relatives.

— Dreams, running.

— Dreams, shooting.

— Dreams, snow.

— Dreams, strangled, of being.

— Dreams, water.

— Dreams, water, bathing.

— Dreams, water, swimming.

— Dullness, sluggishness.

— Dwells on past, disagreeable occurrences.

— Embarrassment.

— Ennui.

— Estranged, friends, from.

— Excitement, excitable, trifles, over.

— Fear, examination, before.

— **Forsaken feeling**.

— Forsaken feeling, beloved by parents, wife, friends, feels, is not being.

— Forsaken feeling, sense of isolation.

— Impatience, hurry.

— Impulse, morbid, run about, to, dromomania.

— Indifference, everything, to.

— Indolence, aversion to work.

— *Irritability*.

— Introspection.

— Irritability, family, to her.

— Irritability, headache, during.

— Loquacity.

— Mistakes, makes, time, in.

— Patient.

— Prostration of mind, mental exhaustion, brain fag.

— Quarrelsomeness, scolding.

— Quarrelsomeness, scolding, family,

with, his or her.

— Remorse.

— Restlessness, nervousness.

— Sadness, melancholy.

— Self-control, wants to control himself.

— Selfishness, egoism.

— Starting, fright, from, and as from.

— Starting, sleep, during.

— Starting, touched, when.

— Striking.

— Succeeds never.

— Talk, indisposed to, desire to be silent, taciturn.

— Thoughts, clearness of.

— Thoughts, rush of

— Thoughts, strangeness of.

— Tranquility.

— Weary of life.

— Weeping, tearful mood.

— Weeping, tearful mood, afternoon, 2 p.m.

— Weeping, tearful mood, causeless.

— *Will, contradiction of*.

— Work, desire for mental.

Physical symptoms

Generalities
- Activity, increased.
- Activity, physical, evening.
- Energy, lots of.
- Exertion, physical, aversion for.
- Food and drink, cold drinks, water, desires.
- Food and drink, cream desires.
- Food and drink, egg desires.
- Food and drink, milk desires.
- Food and drink, rich food desires.
- Food and drink, tea aggravates.
- Food and drink, tea desires.
- Heat, sensation of.
- Lassitude.
- Lie down, inclination to.
- Pain, night.
- Sensitiveness, externally.
- Touch aggravates, slight.
- Weakness.
- Weakness, evening aggravates.
- Weariness.

Vertigo
- Vertigo.
- Morning, rising, on, aggravates.
- Vertigo, accompanied by head, heaviness in the head.
- Vertigo, accompanied by staggering.
- Bed, motion, as if in.
- Fall, tendency to.
- Lying, while, aggravates, side on.
- Lying, while, ameliorates, back on.
- Standing while aggravates.

Head
- Constriction.
- Constriction, forehead.

- Constriction, temples.
- Empty, hollow sensation.
- Eruptions.
- Eruptions, occiput.
- Heaviness.
- Heaviness, afternoon ameliorates (single).
- Heaviness, ascending on.
- **Pain**.
- Pain, accompanied by nausea.
- Pain, air, draft of air.
- Pain, bathing, warm ameliorates (single).
- *Pain, motion, ameliorates.*
- Pain, motion, rapid ameliorates (single).
- Pain, music, from.
- Pain, pressure ameliorates.
- Pain, reading aggravates.
- Pain, riding, cars, on, the.
- Pain, sitting aggravates.
- Pain, walking ameliorates.
- *Pain, forehead.*
- Pain, forehead, eminence, frontal, morning, waking, on.
- Pain, forehead, nose, above root of.
- Pain, occiput.
- Pain, occiput, morning.
- Pain, temples, right.
- Pain, vertex.
- *Pain, dull.*
- Pain, dull, evening ameliorates (single).
- Pain, dull, closing eyes, ameliorates (single).
- Pain, dull, closing eyes, ameliorates.
- Pain, dull, motion, rapid, ameliorates (single).

- Pain, dull, pressure ameliorates.
- Pain, dull, forehead.
- Pain, dull, forehead, morning.
- Pain, dull, forehead, afternoon ameliorates (single).
-- Pain, dull, occiput, extending to sides (single).
- Pain, dull, vertex.
- Pain, pressing, forehead, eyes, over.
- Pain, pressing, forehead, eyes, over, morning.
- Pain, pressing, vertex.
- Pain, shooting, pressure ameliorates.
- Pain, shooting, pulsating.
- Pain, shooting, temples, right.
- Pain, stitching, motion ameliorates.
-- Pain, stitching, pulsating.
- Pain, stitching, occiput, extending to vertex (single).
- Pain, stitching, sides, left.
- Pulsating.
- Pulsating, morning.
- Pulsating, afternoon, 4 p.m.
- Pulsating, light.
- Pulsating, motion aggravates.
- Pulsating, noise, from.
- Pulsating, pressure aggravates (single).
- Pulsating, pressure ameliorates.
- Pulsating, forehead, evening.
- Pulsating, occiput, afternoon.
- Pulsating, sides, left.
- Pulsating, sides, left.
- Pulsating, temples, right.
- Pulsating, vertex, evening (single).

Eyes

- Closing the eyes, desire to.
- Heaviness.

- Heaviness, lids.
- Opening the eyelids, difficult.
- Pain, aching lids, morning, waking, on (single).
- Pain, burning.
- Pain, burning, right.
- Swelling, right.
- Swelling, upper lids, right.

Ear

- Pain, drawing, right.
- Pain, stitching, right.
- Pain, stitching, deaf ear, in.
- Stopped sensation.

Nose

- Catarrh.
- Catarrh, postnasal.
- Coryza.
- Discharge, thick.
- Discharge, viscid, tough.
- Discharge, watery.
- Discharge, white.
- Discolouration, redness, tip.
- Itching, nostrils.
- Obstruction.
- Obstruction, one side.
- Obstruction, right.
- Obstruction, morning, rising, on (single).
- Pain, pressing, nostril, left (single).
- Sneezing.
- Sneezing, morning.
- Sneezing, morning, and evening.
- Sneezing, air draft, in.
- Sneezing, cold air, in.
- Sneezing, constant, morning (single).
- Sneezing, coryza, without.
- Sneezing, paroxysmal.

Face
- Eruptions, cheek, left.
- Eruptions, forehead.
- Eruptions, boils, forehead.
- Eruptions, pimples, forehead.
- Perspiration, mouth, around (single).

Mouth
- Aphtae.
- Bleeding gums.
- Dryness.
- Odour, offensive.
- Pain, burning, palate.
- Pain, stitching, lip, inside of, upper, aphtae, in (single).
- Saliva, offensive.
- Saliva, saltish.
- Salivation, morning, waking, on.

Throat
- Choking.
- Discolouration, redness.
- Dryness.
- Fullness.
- Itching.
- Pain.
- Pain, extending to ears.
- Pain, burning.
- Pain, burning, drinks, warm ameliorate.
- Pain, burning, swallowing, when.
- Pain, sore, coughing, on.
- Pain, stitching, right.
- Pain, stitching, night.
- Tickling.

External throat
- Eruptions, painful.
- Eruptions, red.
- Itching.
- Sprained, sensation.

- Sprained, sensation, lie on back, compelled to (single).
- Sprained sensation, lying side, on, aggravates (single).

Stomach
- Appetite diminished.
- Appetite increased.
- Emptiness, tea, from drinking (single).
- Heaviness.
- Nausea.
- Nausea, food looking at, on.
- Pain, burning.
- Thirst.
- Thirst, night.
- Thirst, large quantities, for, often and.
- Vomiting, food, midnight, 2.30 a.m., waking, on, from a dream of strangulation (single).
- Vomiting, yellow.

Abdomen
- Constriction, sides, left (single).
- Constriction, umbilicus, region, of.
- Distention.
- Eruptions, itching.
- Flatulence.
- Heaviness.
- Itching, inguinal region.
- Pain.
- Pain, morning.
- Pain, laughing aggravates.
- Pain, stool, before.
- Pain, hypogastrium, right.
- Pain, hypogastrium, jarring aggravates.
- Pain, inguinal region.
- Pain, umbilicus.
- Pain, cramping.
- Pain, cutting, pressure ameliorates.

- Pain, cutting, sides, right, left to (single).
- Pain, drawing.
- Tension, evening.

Rectum
- Constipation.
- Constipation, difficult stool.
- Diarrhoea.
- Diarrhoea, morning.
- Pain, burning.
- Pain, tenesmus.
- Pain, tenesmus, midnight, 3.00 a.m. (single).
- Pain, tenesmus, stool before.
- Urging, evening.
- Urging, sudden.

Stool
- Dark.
- Flatulent.
- Forcible, sudden, gushing.
- Frequent.
- Green.
- Lumps, liquid and.
- Mucous.
- Odour, offensive.
- Watery.
- Yellow.

Bladder
- Urination frequent.

Cough
- Morning.
- Night.
- Dry.
- Forcible.
- Paroxysmal.
- Violent.

Expectoration
- Morning.
- Stringy.
- Taste, saltish.
- Thick.
- Viscid.
- Yellow.

Chest
- Discharge from nipple, milky, in male (single).
- Eruptions, axilla right (single).
- Eruptions, axilla, itching.
- Pain, lying.
- Pain, sides, left.
- Pain, heart, region of.
- Pain, heart, region of, evening ameliorates (single).
- Pain, dull, sternum, behind (single).
- Pain, sticking in ribs (single).
- Palpitation, morning, waking, on.

Back
- Itching, evening, bed, in.
- Pain, sitting, long after.
- Pain, lumbar region.

Extremities
- Cramps, upper limbs.
- Cramps, lower limbs.
- *Eruptions, itching*.
- Eruptions, painful.
- Eruptions, elbow, bend of, pimples.
- Eruptions, forearm, red.
- Eruptions, foot, red.
- Eruptions, foot, itching.
- Heat, palms.
- Heaviness, foot.
- Itching, knee, morning, 6 a.m. (single).
- Itching, foot, back of.

- Numbness, hand, fingers, right.
- Numbness, hand, fingers, night midnight after, 4.00-5.00 a.m. (single).
- Numbness, hand, first finger.
- Numbness, hand, second finger.
- Pain, hand, touch, on.
- Pain, hip.
- Pain, knee, hollow of, walking, on.
- Pain, leg.
- Pain, leg, night.
- Pain, leg, motion ameliorates.
- Pain, lower limbs.
- Pain, lower limbs, sitting, while.
- Pain, lower limbs, walking, on.
- Weakness, lower limbs.

Sleep
- *Disturbed.*
- Disturbed, **midnight, after, 3.00 a.m.** (single).
- Falling asleep, **daytime**.

- Falling, late.
- Restless.
- *Sleepiness.*
- Sleepiness, day time.
- Sleepiness, morning.
- Sleepiness, evening.
- Sleepiness, reading.
- *Sleeplessness.*
- Sleeplessness, night, midnight, after, 1.00-2.00 a.m., until.
- Sleeplessness, thoughts, activity of thoughts, from.
- Unrefreshing.
- Waking, anxiety, as from.
- Waking, difficult.
- Waking, frequent.

Chill
- Night, midnight, after, 4.00 a.m.

Skin
- Itching, spots.

THEMES

1. **Two wills**
   Spiritual and God fearing, versus unreligious and sinful.
   Need to improve at work, versus need to relax, go on a holiday, take a break.
   Individuality versus group conformity.

2. **Helping others**
   People weaker or less fortunate (example: handicapped cousin).
   Friend who did not succeed in practice.
   Elderly man.
   People unknown to him.
   People from another, even rival, community
   Patients, sick friends.
   Feeling that I should think of myself first, and then of others.
   Thinking of others rather than of himself.
   Helping even the person (father) who has wronged him.
   Feeling that one should never ever share with others.

3. **Cousins**
   Anxiety for, helping, assisting.
   Quarrelling with.
   Saving from being murdered.

4. **Friends**
   Forsaken, left alone, by.
   Assisting sick friends.
   Quarrelling with.
   Reprimanded by, in her own interest.
   Enjoying the company of.

5. **Family / Relatives**
   Turned out by family.
   Anxiety for relatives.
   Doing things for family (example: treating sick father, despite being wronged).
   Preparing milk-drink for mother, even though she found it difficult.
   Two families living together in the same house.
   Large joint family.

6. **Community**
   Being helped by members of rival community.
   Inter-community riots.

7. **Snakes**
   Fear of.
   Surrounded by.
   Snakes escaping, slippery.
   Criminal being being held in, and escaping.
   Pursued by murderer.

9. Revered person, and middle-aged person making sexual advances.

10. Raping, threatening for revenge.

11. **Uncaring**
    Shooting elderly passer-by, with enjoyment and thrill.
    Borrowing neighbour's car, and not bothering to return it.

12. **Impulses**
    To throttle a teacher.
    To run.
    To beat someone.
    To inflict self-harm.

13. **Conforming**
    Individuality versus group conformity.
    Turned out of house (for example: for failing exams).

Need to be dressed in the presence of others.

Embarrassment, (for example: from odd attire, because of his large appetite).

Being reprimanded by teachers.

Being reprimanded by mother for rude behaviour.

Rituals.

14. Indifference.

15. **Alone / Forsaken**

Alone in the world.

Forsaken by friends, "cut off".

Unloved by family.

Forsaken by aunt to whom she was very close.

Left alone by husband.

"Isolated" feeling.

Loving someone only causes you pain.

16. **Despair**

Can't do anything bright in the future.

Desires death.

Suicidal thoughts from the feeling that no one understands him.

17. **Disgust**

About oneself, one's diseased body.

18. Laboured effort.

Discovering a new place.

Adventure.

Unravelling a mystery.

Achieving something better, teaching students better and desiring the progress of his science.

To overtake everyone else.

Small boy escaping from captivity to become a great monk.

19. **Large houses**

Land.

Car.

Money.

Friend had two pianos, while she had none.

20. **Journeys**

Deserted road.

Curved road.

Road with many ups and downs.

Long train journey from Bombay to London.

21. **Floods**

Warning others about floods.

Making social call in spite of floods.

22. **Pursued**

Women pursued by men.

Animals, by.

Murderer, by.

23. **Danger**

Fire.

Accident.

Death.

24. **Old, deserted palace**

Ruined fort.

25. Assembly of people appreciating an honest man

26. Tyrant.

27. Experiment on human beings.

28. Small man.

Large men fitting into small suitcases.

29. Sadness, weeping.

Taciturn

30. **Irritability, quarrelsomeness**

31. **Restlessness, impatience, hurry**

7

THE PROVING OF *LAC LEONINUM*

I conducted a proving of *Lac leoninum* in March 1994. Six provers, including myself, participated. They were between the ages of twenty and thirty-five years old. Prover F did not take the dose.

During the first meeting the provers were given doses of the substance in the 30 C potency with instruction to take first a single dose, and watch for symptoms. In case they did not get any symptoms, they were advised to take subsequent doses. The provers met me individually at the end of every week, over the following three weeks. After the third week, we met as a group, discussed the proving and I revealed the name of the substance to them. If they had any further symptoms, they were asked to continue to keep in touch with me and report the same. These symptoms have also been incorporated into the proving.

The drug was prepared as follows:
- Milk that had been obtained from a lactating lioness was triturated upto the 3 C potency using a mortar and pestle. Further potencies were prepared by hand, in alcohol by the Hahemannian method.

Emotions

Irritability / Anger

▪ Very irritable and impatient. Very sensitive, easily offended. Imagined admonitions and "fired" back. Felt that people were trying to put me down, blame me, find fault with me, criticize me. Became tearful from this. Felt that they were making me feel inferior or low. Began "firing" back, and putting others down. Later, apologized for my behaviour.

[C/f/1,*/iii]

▪ Agitated at slight things, irritable. Expressed irritability which I usually suppress; was happy to do it. Felt how dare people tell me these things for no fault of mine; they had no right to. Advised an aunt not to let people to take advantage, and to give back, shrewdly, and teach others a lesson.

[B/f/2,*/i]

▪ Anger, offended, ego hurt. Took a pledge not to visit the offender again. Felt she should come to me rather than me go to her.

[B/f*,*/*]

▪ Expressed anger towards a woman who was constantly instructing me.

[A/f/2,*,*/i]

▪ Anger at interference.

[B/f/1,*/i]

▪ Very irritable and quarrelsome from interference in my matters. Flared up, and had a desire to smash my brother who I felt was interfering, but controlled myself. Wanted my independence. Felt it was my life and he had no right to interfere.

[E/f/1,*/*]

▪ Irritability, desire to strike those who pester me constantly.

[E/f/2,*/*]

▪ Felt I wanted to crash the face of people who stared at me.

[A/f/2,*/*]

▪ Over-reacted when I thought my servant was being haughty, too dominating and trying to point out my mistake. Was boiling with anger and had the malicious plan of removing her from my service. Started to talk behind her back, but did not confront her. At one point when she made a complaint, it got too much and I exploded. Called everyone and told them about it. How dare she! Abused her. Felt that even my husband was taking her side. I gave him an ultimatum that either I would stay in the house or the servant. Wanted to get rid of her. Could not tolerate her domination. Wouldn't allow it. Would jump at husband, pounce upon him, quarrel with him to make her leave. I felt that they were all trying to show that I was inferior and foolish and that I had to give back and fight at any cost, insult them. Fretted and fumed. Decided that if I didn't win, I would get out.

[C/f/2,*/iv]

Hindered

▪ Feeling as if someone was trying to

create a problem for me but I had to struggle and get over it. While I am determined to fight the problem by hook or by crook, I am also feeling attacked. I am oversensitive and easily offended. Feel as if others want to show that I am inferior, and want to run away when I feel that the criticism gets too much. Want to retaliate, but not interested in patching up at any cost.

[C/f/2,*/iv]

- Felt that others were being selfish and not letting me experience things.

[C/f/1,*/iii]

Confidence

- Lack of confidence to speak and express myself in front of elderly, respected persons. Imagine that people are laughing at me.

[D/m/1,2/i]

- Feeling weak, fragile, lonely. Timid, as if I have to depend on others for everything. Wanted a friend to solve a problem of mine.

[E/f/2,*/*]

Behaviour

- Blaming others.

[B/f/1,*/i]

- Outrageous, uncivilized behaviour. Pouncing and jumping on others as soon as they told me anything.

[B/f/2,*/ii]

- Loud voice.

[B/f/2,*/ii]

- Blunt speech, uncaring for the feelings of others.

[B/f/2,*/ii]

- Abrupt, harsh, outspoken.

[C/f/1,*/iii]

- Vehemently assertive attitude.

[C/f/2,*/iv]

- Depression, scolding on waking.

[E/f/2,*/*]

Activity

- Restlessness, changing places frequently. Want to move about.

[E/f/1,*/*]

- Desire to do many things, but my body does not assist me; prostrated.

[E/f/2,*/*]

- Energetic with an inclination to do many things that had been pending.

[C/f/1,*/iii]

- Desire to constantly buy new, different, and good clothes in various shades of red.

[E/f/2,*/*]

- Desire to go out of the house, don't want to stay at home.

[E/f/2,*/*]

Miscellaneous

- Singing and desire to dance on waking in the morning, without the tension I had been feeling about the forthcoming exams.

[E/f/1,1/*]

- Felt very strong and great like a king, and thought of others that they were slow creatures who were in my way.

[A/f/1,*/i]

- Clairvoyance.

[B/f/before dose]

- An unnecessary anxiety about domestic problems.

[C/f/1,*/iii]

- Excited and eager to do my best to help relatives in an emergency situation.

[C/f/1,*/iii]

- Was very impressed with a woman I have known and began to compare her with every other woman I know. I aspired to be like her, and was also motivating my mother in the same direction. About the woman:

She is very modern in her way of dressing and her ideas; a very forward personality, an extrovert. She likes to go for concerts and parties, and does not want to be sitting at home doing the same thing.

She is married to a businessman and although she is not very highly educated, her husband has come up because of her. She helps him in his factory, and attends and conducts business conferences with a lot of confidence. In spite of being only a graduate she deals with engineers and even designs machinery, handles production and marketing herself. She once conducted a meeting with the managers of several well-known firms in which she was on the top, bossing over, convincing and impressing everyone (her husband who was also present sat in a corner without being able to do anything).

Although she appears very posh, she is not a snob, in fact she is very sweet-natured, and yet she can convince anyone in a split second. She could sell an old diary or perhaps even a broken object very convincingly. She is very flattering and speaks what-

ever the other person wants her to.

She is attractive and charming, even though she does not have a good figure in the conventional sense of the word; she is in fact "built up". But she looks after herself, has beautiful hair and complexion, and can be quite seductive. I felt she is everything a woman should be.

I felt of her that she is next to Mrs. Indira Gandhi[1] with the same look, confident talk and leadership qualities. I was attracted and allured by her craving for power. She gains power by appearing modest and adopting a low profile.

She is constantly in demand at any function of social importance –whether it be a party, a conference or a concert, and is always the centre of attraction there, is never in the background.

[E/f/1,*/*]

---

[1]   Former Indian Prime Minister.

DREAMS

Left out / Alone / Uncared for

• A fine lady was riding in an elegant, black car (like a Porsche or a Jaguar) without any windows or driver, through a Bombay street. She was white-skinned, and had red hair of shoulder length. She was in severe agony, was tossing her head from one side to another and I knew that she had sepsis. A local person said to me that they did not wish to have her in their area. I wondered as to why they were treating such a fine lady below her standard. It was like they drove her out, did not look after her.

[A/f/1,*/*]

• One out of four girls who were modelling is not selected, and asked modestly to

go out. Felt depressed and taciturn on waking from the dream.

[E/f/1,3/*]

• My best friend had patched up with her boyfriend after a fight despite my telling her that he wasn't a good person, and that she wouldn't be happy with him. I felt angry, left out and all alone because she did not listen to me. Also, I was concerned that he was selfish and would break up with her once again.

[E/f/1,*/*]

• I had a child who was supposed to be mine, but born out of a marriage with a woman I did not love. At birth, he had an abscess in the left side of his chest, which had formed a fistula that was oozing dirty pus. The abcess had been covered with a bandage. Then I realized that the child had been conceived with the sperm of another man and the ovum of a strange woman, which had been fertilized in the womb of another woman. So I felt that this was not my child. But even if it had been, it was not born out of love. I had no desire to care for it and left it in the care of my aunt, with the feeling that he would not survive. But somehow he did survive, and was left with a dark, black eruption on the right side of his chest.

[F'/m/1,1/0]

Danger

▪ We had to go on a ship, though I knew it was dangerous and we would die. As we were driving towards it, I felt that I was quite big, but when we were overtaken by some huge people, I felt quite small in comparison to them. Coming from the opposite direction were some strange, spider-like figures, like out of the movie, "Dinosaur"; I felt they were interesting and exciting, rather than fearful.

I was worried because we had to find our way though the trees. Then we came to the seashore where the ship was waiting. There were many people on it, and I knew that they would die and only the best would survive. There seemed to be a "fitting test" in store.

There were attempts to persuade us to get on board by people who were friendly, and who were promising us many things. But I knew that once we got onto the ship the trouble would start. Everything around us that we touched or smelled was polluted... the grass, the meadows. There was a lion there that belonged to those trying to persuade us, and beyond the lion was a beautiful meadow to charm us. I wanted, desperately, to warn the others of the dangers ahead, and to tell them not to be charmed. But there was no escape, we had no choice. We would have

to follow in spite of knowing what dangers lay ahead.

[A/f/2,*/*]

▪ My father had been beaten up by many persons because he had witnessed a murder. He was in a pool of blood and came running home. He packed our bags and urged us to leave, saying we would be killed if we stayed. We ran away to an undisclosed destination, closed the door of the house we were in, and stayed indoors. We did not go to church even though it was a Sunday. Then someone rang the bell and my mother wanted to answer the door but I stopped her, saying that if someone was going to be killed, let me be the first one. On opening the door, we were relieved to find that it was only the parish priest.

Regarding the priest:

He is six-feet tall, heavily built (about 120 kg), keeps his hair and beard long, wears glasses.

Unlike other Christian priests who wear cassocks, he wears saffron robes like a sannyasi [1] even when conducting a mass. People call him "Swamiji" [2]. He is very much like a sannyasi, has "mukti" (is liberated) from everything and does not believe in relationships.

He had once met with an accident, and the eye of a goat was transplanted for his lost eye. He brought education into our community and made us progress. He works with alcoholics, looks after and educates their families. He doesn't talk too much, but only meaningful things. He comes to us whenever something goes wrong or if we are in trouble and prays for us. He also comes at auspicious moments, and when we want to do something good.

---

[1]   Hindu saint.
[2]   Hindu ascetic.

He is well-known in the entire region of South West Maharashtra.

[E/f/1,1/*]

▪ I was in a lonely house and wanted to shut all the windows to be safe from robbers, but wanted also the sunlight to come in and so I couldn't keep everything shut. I was wondering how to be safe.

[A/f/2,*/*]

Animals

▪ We were admiring a nice, old house with a big garden and many hills all around. It belonged to an old lady. As I looked at the roughly cut lawn, I thought that once it had been a nice English lawn. I said that as a child I would have wanted to just lie in bed and look down at the lawn. Then we saw strange, large, tall and muscular creatures with faces like monkeys. We knew they were dangerous and went inside the house, but my father went outside to the monkeys.

The monkeys were trying to get into the house and we began to shut the windows. One managed to get in before I could shut a window. I felt I needed to fight back or take some action and hit him on both sides of the eyes with a big log of wood. Then I wondered if he was really dead, and picked up the skull and saw the brain beneath. I felt superior and bigger. Another girl also managed to kill a monkey. We managed to get them out of the house.

Once again we began to shut all the doors and windows; it was night time and my father returned. We were happy that we had room, and that my father was safe.

[A/f/2,*/*]

▪ My younger cousin was weeping, crying to be taken outdoors. There were tigers and bears in the forest outside. A tiger began to pursue us. I sent the child indoors first,

and managed to get indoors myself just before it pounced upon me. I was fearful of being killed, feeling I was all alone to save myself and my cousin.

[E/f/2,*/*]

▪ The face of a tiger or a lion when a person opened his mouth.

[A/f/1,*/*]

▪ A very small pet lion which bit my finger and jumped on to me when I let it out of its cage. It ran under the sofa, but I caught it and put it back in its cage, though I knew it could not escape.

[A/f/2,*/*]

▪ A small mouse was chasing a big cat.

[E/f/1,*/*]

▪ A doctor of various personalities takes us to a dark attic for a lesson. There are many papers there and a grey-black, hefty cat who won't go even though my friend tries a lot to "shoo" her off. Finally the doctor manages to get rid of the cat.

[B/f/2,*/*]

Deceiving / Bribing / Cheating

▪ I was sitting in the corridor of my very huge house when a brahmin (hindu priest) came to me asking for monetary help, and saying that he was lost. I became very angry because I felt he was trying to cheat me, and arrogantly gave him the names of two-three social service institutions that help brahmins. I felt guilty because I knew I could have helped him, although I had not wanted to.

Later, I was telling my compounder that one should be aware that people try and cheat you. I felt I was just trying to cover up for my feeling of guilt.

[D/m/1,1/i]

▪ My best friend (male) who is very sexual-minded, a young beautiful virgin girl and myself are together in my bedroom, naked, with the intention of sexual intercourse. We are all unmarried, and are very eager. Like them, I too regard the whole idea

---

¹ Western Indian State of which Bombay is the Capital city.

(which I normally do not like nor accept, but which has always been my best friend's fantasy), as fun. My best friend is giving me the first chance. The only hindrance is a blind man (clothed) who is also present in the room. We do not want him there; he may come to know our secret. I take him to another room under some pretext. Later, he asks me for something to eat and I take him to kitchen and give him some left-overs.

[D/m/1,5/ii]

- Getting over a hurdle which is in the way of doing something, satisfying someone, by giving a bribe.

[D/m/2,*/*]

- There has been a murder and the police have come to inspect the body. They do not allow anyone to see it except for one girl who has paid them some money.

[E/f/1,1/*]

Offended / Ego hurt

- I am wearing dark goggles in the morning. A friend does not recognize me. I feel I should call out to her, but don't. My ego is hurt.

[B/f/1,*/*]

- I am going far away in a bullock-cart because I was offended.

[C/f/2,*/iv]

- I was visited by my cousin who had hurt my ego. I answered her in monosyllables.

[B/f/1,*/*]

Friends

- I am attending to a library, when a school friend comes and asks for a book called "Face Value". I give her a novel but she refuses it and takes a magazine of the same name. I feel bad, and am embarrassed.

[B/f/1,*/*]

- My friends and me were not being allowed to stand in a queue by some other people.

[B/f/ before dose]

- School friends.

[B/f/1,5/i]

- I convince a school friend to buy a pink rose from my shop. After she leaves, surprisingly, another pink rose turns to brown, and I am a little concerned as to what she will think of me if her pink rose becomes brown as well.

[B/f/2,*/*]

- A friend wants to share a taxi with me since we are going to the same destination. I do not want to go with her because I get the bad feeling that I will not reach. But I go all the same. The taxi driver takes many wrong turns before we finally reach our destination and I am relieved to find a familiar person there.

[B/f/1,*/*]

- My friends were angry with me because I had forgotten to wear traditional clothes to college on the occasion of a traditional day.

[E/f/1,2/*]

- While I was taking the case of a very close friend, a classmate came and said of her that her eyes are very big and that she was dangerous. We laughed together.

[B/f/2,*/*]

Miscellaneous

- We were going in a dark bus on a mountainous route and I was wondering how I got there.

[B/f/ before dose]

- A dark face, presumably my own, with hair pulled apart, calling out in agony, misery, frustration.

[C/f/2,*/iv]

- I was in a dance lesson which was being taken by a teacher. I did not like. It was very accurately arranged and she would give us notes later, but I was very clumsy and felt very stupid somehow.

[A/f/2,*/*]

- My professor was telling me not to attend subsequent lectures because I hadn't attended his previous lectures.

[E/f/1,2/*]

- Making a business deal regarding some property.

[E/f/1,2/*]

- I am refusing to allow other colleagues to sit in with me for a case, even though a teacher has sent them. They want to join in just when I am probing a very sensitive point in the patient's history.

[B/f/1,*/*]

- Film star.

[B/f/1,*/*]

- A yellow, cheezy mass in my throat was suffocating me. It was bloating up, puffing up and I could not breathe (woke up with pus in the throat and difficulty in breathing).

[A/f/before dose]

- A taxi driver who is cruel and cunning, is telling a prostitute that he will get her customers. I think to myself: "The bastard! He is doing this sort of business as well!"

[D/m/1,3/i]

- I was hanging onto a bar which was similar to a pole-vault and some fifty feet above the ground. There was a second similar bar at a distance and I wanted to swing from one bar to the other, but found it impossible, the distance between them being too great.

Later I was swinging on a swing that was similar to those one sees in a circus.

[D/m/1,1/i]

- I am directing my compounder who is swinging on horizontal bars.

[D/m/1,2/i]

PHYSICAL SYMPTOMS

Generalities

- Tiredness and sluggishness.
[B/f/before dose]

- Inability to tolerate hunger.
[C/f/1,*/iii]

- Desire for pungent food.
[C/f/2,*/iv]

- Sore, bruised, aching pains on waking in the morning.
[E/f/1,2/*]

- Tiredness, mental and physical.
[E/f/1,*/*]

- Heaviness.
[B/f/1,*/*]

- Malaise.
[B/f/1,*/*]

- Morning aggravation.
[B/f/1,*/*]

- Unable to bear heat.
[B/f/1,*/*]

- Desire for open air.
[E/f/2,*/*]

- Morning aggravates, evening ameliorates.
[E/f/2,*/*]

Physical particulars

Head

• Frontal heaviness and pain, aggravated in the morning.

[B/f/1,*/*]

Eyes

• Constant blinking of left eye.

[B/f/ before dose]

• Burning heat in the eyes.

[B/f/1,*/*]

Throat

• Sensation of something stuck in the throat, troubling me.

[B/f/1,*/*]

Stomach

• Intense nausea, aggravated in the morning.

[B/f/1,*/*]

• Decreased appetite, a few mouthfuls fill up.

[E/f/1,*/*]

Abdomen

• Severe stitching pain in groin and right renal region.

[A/f/1,*/*]

• Sensation of fullness, bloatedness.

[E/f/1,2/*]

• Pain in the hypogastrium as at the onset of menses.

[B/f/1,*/*]

Urinary organs

• Irritation in the initial part of urination.

[C/f/2,*/iv]

Cough

• Cough – spasmodic, aggressive.

[A/f/2,*/*]

Extremities

• Itching in the forearm.

[C/f/2,*/iv]

• Violently itching, raised eruptions beginning on forearm and the back of the thigh, with burning stinging pains; scratching.

[B/f/1,*/*]

• Severe pain in legs as if I would tear off the skin, unable to stand long.

[E/f/2,*/*]

Sleep

• Sleepiness from sitting in one place. Must change places constantly.

[E/f/1,*/*]

• Sleepiness throughout the day.

[B/f/1,*/*]

RUBRICS

Mind

Single symptoms
— Admonitions aggravate, imagined.
— *Anger, interference at.*
— Assertive, vehemently.
— Clothes, desires red.
— Dancing, morning, waking, on.
— Delusion experiences things she was not allowed to, selfish, those around her were, because.
— Delusion, king, she is.
— *Delusion, put down, she is.*
— Dreams, agony, of being in.
— Dreams, animals, monkeys, trying to get into her house.
— Dreams, animals, mouse, small, pursuing a big cat.
— Dreams, arrogant, of being.
— Dreams, bigger and superior, of being.
— Dreams, cheating, suspicious, of being cheated.
— Dreams, child with abcess on chest oozing dirty pus.
— Dreams, cruel and cunning person.
— Dreams, driven out, being.
— Dreams, father, being beaten.
— Dreams, friends forsaken by her.
— Dreams, face, dark, with hair pulled apart, calling out in agony.
— Dreams, guilty for refusing charity.
— Dreams, hindered, of being.
— Dreams, house, huge.
— Dreams, house, lonely, being, in a.
— Dreams, journeys, mountainous region, in a.
— Dreams, killed, she volunteers to be the first one to be killed.
— Dreams, murder, witnessing a.
— Dreams, people, huge.
— *Dreams, pride hurt.*
— Dreams, pursued, saving a child from a pursuing tiger.
— Dreams, secret sexuality.
— Dreams, swinging, bars, from, he was.
— Dreams, windows, she had to shut, to be safe.
— Dreams, woman, dangerous, big eyes, with.
— Dreams, woman, fine, being treated below her standard.
— Interference, intolerance of, self-control must exercise, violent impulses, over.
— *Intolerance, domination, of.*
— Malicious, uncompromising.
— *Pounce or jump at others, desire to.*
— Quarrelsomeness, scolding, morning, waking, on.

Common symptoms
— Abrupt.
— Abusive.
— Ailments, from honour, wounded.
— Ailments, from indignation.
— **Anger, irrascibility**.
— Anger, besides himself.
— *Anger, violent.*
— Answers, abruptly.
— Answers, civil, cannot be.
— Answers, monosyllables, in.
— Answers, snappishly.
— Anxiety, household, matters about.

— Change, desire for.
— Clairvoyance.
— Confidence, want of self.
— Contemptuous.
— Deceitful, sly.
— Delusion, attacked, being.
— Delusion, criticized, she is.
— Delusion, fragile.
— Delusion, great person, he is.
— Delusion, hindered, he is, everyone, by.
— Delusion, laughed at, mocked, being.
— Delusion, persecuted.
— Delusion, strong, he is.
— Dreams, amorous.
— *Dreams, animals, wild.*
— *Dreams, danger.*
— Dreams, danger, death, of.
— Dreams, insects, of.
— Dreams, embarrassment.
— *Dreams, friends, old.*
— Dreams, movie star (*Dendroaspis polylepsis, Coca-Cola*).
— Dreams, journey, of.
— Dreams, murder.
— Dreams, pursued, animals, by, wild.
— Egotism, self-esteem.
— Escape, attempts to.

— *Fight, wants to.*
— Forsaken feeling.
— Hard-hearted.
— Haughty.
— *Impatience.*
— Impolite.
— Impulse, morbid, violence to do .
— Indignation.
— Intolerance.
— **Irritability**.
— Irritability, trifles, at.
— Malicious.
— Offended easily.
— Power, love, of.
— *Quarrelsomeness, scolding.*
— Rage, fury.
— Reproaches others.
— Restlessness, move about constantly, must.
— Sadness, morning, waking, on.
— Sensitive, oversensitive, reprimands, criticism, reproaches, to.
— Singing, morning, waking, on.
— Striking, desire, strike, to.
— Sympathetic.
— Threatening.
— Timidity.
— Unsympathetic.

PHYSICAL SYMPTOMS

Generalities
– *Morning.*
– Evening ameliorates.
– Air, open, desire for.
– Food, desires, pungent.
– Heaviness.

– Hunger aggravates.
– Pain, sore, bruised, morning, waking, on.
– Sluggishness of the body.
– Warm aggravates.
– *Weakness.*

Head
- Heaviness, forehead, morning.
- Pain, forehead, morning.

Eye
- Heat, in.
- Twitching, lids, left.
- Winking.

Throat
- Foreign body, sensation of.
- Lump, sensation.

Stomach
- Appetite, easy satiety.
- Appetite, wanting.
- Nausea, morning.

Abdomen
- Distention.
- Fullness, sensation of.
- Pain, hypogastrium.
- Pain, stitching, inguinal region.
- Pain, stitching, sides, right.

Urethra
- Irritation.

Larynx
- Voice loud.

Cough
- Paroxysmal.
- Spasmodic.
- Violent.

Extremities
- Eruptions, forearm, itching.
- Eruptions, forearm, urticaria.
- Eruptions, thigh, burning.
- Eruptions, thigh, itching.
- Eruptions, thigh, urticaria.
- Eruptions, thigh, back of (single).
- *Itching, forearm*.
- Pain, leg.
- Pain, leg, standing.

Sleep
- Sleepiness, daytime.
- Sleepiness, sitting.

THEMES

1.   Feeling that others were putting her down, trying to show that she was inferior and foolish.

Feeling that she was being wrongly blamed, criticized.

Feeling that others were interfering in her life.

Feeling that she was being treated below her standard.

Feeling that others were being selfish, and not letting her experience things.

Feeling that others were taking advantage of her.

Feeling that he was being laughed at.

Feeling that she was weak, fragile, timid, and had to depend on others.

Feeling of being neglected, forsaken.

Feeling that he was hindered; that others put obstacles in her way.

Feeling of being attacked, beaten up.

Feeling of danger.

Feeling that others were trying to cheat him; that they were trying to trap her deceitfully.

Feeling as if there were robbers around, and she was alone against them.

Feeling that her independence was threatened.

2.   Anger with violent impulses. Desire to smash to strike.

Firing, punching those she imagined were attacking, admonishing her, interfering in her life.

Vehemently assertive.

Quarrelsome.

Malicious.

Loud.

Rude, uncivil behaviour.

3.   **Egotism**
Ego hurt.
Love of power.

4.   **Sympathy, caring**
Wanting to help relatives, protect younger cousin.
Parish priest who arrives in a time of need.
Domestic anxiety.

5.   Desire to do many things: restless, but easily prostrated.

6.   **Animals, pursued by**
Being pursued.
Caged.
Attacking her, and she has to defend herself.

7.   **Old friends – neglecting her**
Being offended by.
Afraid to offend.

8.   Small, sick child born out of a loveless marriage, being neglected.

9.   Agony.

10.   Sexuality.

11.   Deceit, cheating, bribing.

12.   Models, film stars.

13.   Clothes in various shades of red.

14.   Singing, dancing.

8

A PROVING OF *NICCOLUM*

The proving of *Niccolum* was conducted in January 1994. The provers, eighteen in number, included participants at the course for foreign students of that year, apart from the usual group of provers. The participants were each given one dose of the substance in the 30 C potency, and were asked to note their symptoms over the next week. Prover J did not take the dose at all, while prover E took it on the third day of the proving. The following week, they met as a group with the master prover. Each of them reported their symptoms and experiences during the week, and at the end of the meeting the proving was discussed. They were asked to continue to note any more symptoms, if any, and to report the same to the master prover; these have also been incorporated into the proving.

The drug was obtained from the pharmacy, "Roy and Company", Bombay.

MIND

Emotions

Anger / Irritability

- Was very angry and "wild" when a person spat betel nut[1] at my feet from a running bus. Got into the bus – wanted to take him to the police. But was unable to find him. Was upset the entire day as a result.

[C/f/1,3/i]

- Was excessively irritable – couldn't tolerate my friends wasting time.

[G/m/1,1/i]

- Felt ditched, cheated, was so angry, so "wild" when a friend, who had forced me to accompany her to a party, was unable to come herself. Fought with her – how could she do this to me! Was irritable.

[C/f/1,2/i]

- Calmness, not affected by emotions. Later, a lot of irritability. Could not tolerate light and noise.

[I/m/1,3/i]

Impulses

- Angry (at a taxi driver), was about to hit him.

[I/m/1,4/i]

- Very angry at a taxi driver who was going the wrong way in spite of repeated instructions. Wanted to wring his neck for being so stupid and unable to understand where I wanted to go.

---

1. A common addiction amonst Indians; leaves a dark red stain, often indelible.

Was also angry at bystanders who were trying to be helpful.

[J'/m/*,*/0]

- Had the sudden impulse, while riding in a taxicab, to put my knife into the back of the taxi driver, and also to cut up the back seat of his cab. There were no feelings associated with the impulse. Later, was very upset and angry when the taxi driver couldn't find the place I wanted to go to.

[K/m/1,3/i]

- Restrained an impulse to be nasty when I was contradicted by someone junior to me; felt he is egoistic and inexperienced.

[A/m/2,*/i]

- Intolerance of contradiction, I felt I was right. Felt like hitting, and did hit one person who couldn't understand my views. Was argumentative, more "debating power"; my friends noted that I was more "dynamic".

[G/m/1,1/i]

Critical / Contemptuous

- Was critical and nasty towards students who came up with suggestions at the end of a case. Told them that I was in a fowl very critical mood (I am normally tolerant).

[A/m/2,*/i]

- Felt about a group of students that they were thick and stupid, when they could not answer a question their teacher had put to them.

[Q/f/*,*/i]

- Was very upset and angry when a waiter took a long time to understand what I wanted; repeatedly told friends about how stupid he had been. We were all really angry.
  [L/f/*,*/i]

- Frustration when a waiter didn't understand and serve us on time. Felt he was stupid, and wondered how anyone could be that "thick". Wanted to complain to the manager.
  [Q/f/*,*/i]

Alternations

- Sudden alternations of mood from joyful to sad.
  [O/f/1,4/i]

- A feeling of being in total control (adult-like), alternating with a feeling of being totally out of control (child-like).
  [A/m/*,*/i]

Activity

- Desire for physical exercise, for example vigorous walking, but found difficulty in walking.
  [A/m/*,*/i]

- Activity increased till afternoon. Then, aversion to physical activity, desire to lie down.
  [O/f/1,1/i]

Weeping / Low mood

- No desire to talk with anyone, was feeling unwanted. Couldn't tolerate sitting alone; wanted to join my group, but didn't want that I should go to them. Got up and left, angry. Felt that nobody wanted me, and felt like dying.

   Was cross and irritable with everyone throughout the day. Was cross, averse to talking especially with my fiancé. Felt only if I could be alone and cry. Later went home and wept alone for half an hour. which relieved. Then regretted my behaviour towards my fiancé, and was feeling that I had made

him suffer.
  [O/f/1,3/i]

- Felt lonely and neglected. Wept in the afternoon. Ameliorated in the evening.
  [O/f/1,4/i]

- Felt low; didn't feel like doing anything.
  [G/m/*,*/i]

- Sensitive, weeping easily.
  [C/f/1,2/i]

Miscellaneous

- Felt very protective towards a female colleague who was going home at a late hour. Felt she had been foolish to have stayed so late. Insisted on dropping her home, although she lived very far away. I imagined she would be attacked by men if she travelled alone at that hour.
  [A/m/1,2/i]

- Anxiety while doing a live-case as to whether I will be able to complete it; the time seemed too little, too narrow.
  [A/m/foll. discussion]

- Was rude in speaking with patients.
  [G/m/1,1/i]

- Feeling of tranquility and peace. Also talked much less.
  [I/m/1,3/i]

- For a few seconds felt lost (while listening to religious songs), as if I was away from this world.
  [I/m/1,4/i]

- Had the feeling that everyone around me was selfish.
  [C/f/1,2/i]

- Talkative and cheerful.
  [K/m/1,1/i]

- Cheerful mood and singing at midnight.
  [K/m/1,1/i]

- Obstinacy.
  [O/f/1,1/i]

- Suspiciousness.

[O/f/1,1/i]

- Vivid fantasies of birds and animals on closing eyes, before falling asleep.

[K/m/1,2/i]

- Had the feeling that my capped tooth had broken with a cracking sound, only to see that nothing had actually happened.

[A/m/*,*/i]

Intellect

- Confusion of mind.

[C/f/1,2/i]

- Lack of concentration.

[C/f/1,3/i]

DREAMS

Attack

- A person jumped out from a tall building into a pond with two alligators in it. They were coming to kill him, and so he took out his knife and killed them.

[E/f/1,2/i]

- I was travelling by train, and missed getting off at my station. I got off at the next station and travelled back. As I was leaving, two men followed me and passed an obscene comment. I took a stick and hit them both.

[E/f/1,2/i]

- While discussing the proving one prover narrated a dream about a frog. I got up and told the master prover that he was bluffing. The prover got angry and kicked me in my abdomen.

[E/f/1,3/i]

Protecting

- I was with my parents and my grandmother (who is dead) at a religious function. There were a cow and goat running around the place. I was protecting my grandmother from the cow, was searching for something with which to keep the cow away.

[P/m/1,1/i]

- I was driving through Madras [1]. I did not know the way. I came across a political procession, and my car was stuck in the crowd. There was a foreign woman with me and I was afraid that the crowd would harm her. I felt protective towards her. Then I started to walk away from the procession towards what turned out to be a police station. Suddenly it seemed I was a foreigner and was in danger from violent persons. I saw a policeman beat a man on the head. I entered the police station and asked the inspector for directions to the place I wanted to reach. He showed me a map.

[A/m/*,*/i]

- I am going into a dark room which belongs to some friends. I am being accompanied by another friend. There are ladies in the house and there is some danger from outside, from which I feel I have to protect the ladies.. We are trying to send a rope ahead so that others can hide.

[A/m/foll. discussion]

- I was travelling on a ship. A man was lighting a match. I was angry at him because

---

[1]   South Indian city.

it was a dangerous thing to do; the ship could catch fire and everyone's lives would be in danger. I felt that the man was stupid and did not know what he was doing.

Then I saw two boys run up the stairs in play. I was very anxious at seeing them and wanted to catch them and protect them. Then one of them fell into the sea.

[N/m/∗,∗/i]

▪ I am bordering a premises that I own with thorny trees, keeping place only for an entrance so that no one can enter it when I play cricket. I am asking my friend to give me some trees.

[B/m/∗,∗/i]

Helping

▪ I am sitting at a window, may be of a train. There is milk powder coming in through the window. A beggar is trying to collect it but is unable to. I start to collect it using a small spoon, which I keep in the direction opposite to the flow of the wind. Then I think I am being foolish and change the direction of the spoon. But since I am not able to collect much with a spoon, I use a box. After it has been filled with the milk powder, I give it to the beggar.

[H/m/1,3/i]

▪ I was going to the beach with friends. We didn't know the way. We were going in the direction opposite to the beach. A person guided us, showed us the way to the beach.

When we got there I was hit by a ball from some boys playing cricket.

[C/f/1,1/i]

▪ I was cycling with my friends, and felt tired after a distance but did not give up. On either side of the road we saw shrivelled up children with tear-filled eyes. We picked them up and put them on a sledge which was attached to our bicycles. A few people asked us while we were cycling, where we were taking the children. We replied that we were

taking them to Mother Theresa's mission.

[R/m/∗,∗/i]

Police

▪ Was in a taxi; the driver was a cheat, he had the meter running too fast. I noticed it and threatened that I would take him to the police. He pushed a button and the meter began to work at its normal pace. Even then, I wanted to take him to the police. I made him park in a lane next to a police station to which I went without his knowledge. The inspector there made a plan, and we got together ropes, jelly and scissors, so that we could tie up the cabbie's hands. I wondered how we would explain this if the he were to ask what we were carrying. The inspector suggested that I tell him that it was for a patient. He accompanied me in plain clothes, and together we nabbed the cabbie. I knew the cabbie could be dangerous but felt I had to do this.

[A/m/1,1/i]

▪ I witness my brother killing my sister. I ask my mother to contact the police. She refuses, saying that it is our family problem and that we cannot disgrace our family by calling in the police. She says that we will just say that it was an accident. But I feel very angry, and want her to tell the truth.

[E/f/1,2/i]

Injustice

▪ I was to go on a train journey with my family. We missed the train by just one minute but were told that we could travel using the same ticket on the next day.

Then we were on the train and I met all my friends there. I offered my seat to a female friend. I saw a poster in the train which read, "Please help unescorted children".

I stood in the doorway and could see four buildings. There were some men standing in the premises. One of them (apparently a builder) was saying to the other that he could mint a lot of money with this land. They rejoiced happily when another man asked about the people who lived in the already existing buildings. He was told that they could just be shifted back into the hutments where they had lived before. I felt that this is injustice.

[I/m/1,2/i]

- I am living in a village house with my family. My father has married a second time. He is sleeping on the bed and has covered himself. My mother is cooking and looks anxious. I see her face and get very angry with my father, thinking about the wrong and injustice that he has done to my mother.

I also see a neighbour outside my house. I feel he is a bad man. I feel angry towards my father and want to tell him that he always blames his sons that they are doing nothing in life, but on the other hand he has neighbours like these.

[H/m/2,6/i]

Water

- Was trying to drive up the steep bank of a beach but could not; was slipping back, more and more into the water. Then the water started to rise and enter the car.

[J'/m/*,*/0]

- I am riding on a bicycle up a hill with my wife on the back seat. Half way up the hill the road is flooded with water. The road has a narrow part I have to go through. If I lose control, I will fall down the hill. I manage to go up, but there is so much water that I have to turn back.

[A/m/*,*/i]

- A very huge water project has been started. It is being broadcast on television. The water level is rising everywhere. A government official is being questioned about the need for the project; he says it is for a better future. I think of my grandmother who had died; she used to be very hot (thermal modality), and would have been uncomfortable.

[P/m/1,2/i]

Miscellaneous

- I had drunk lemon juice at a wayside stall. While paying for it I realized that I had asked for orange juice. I told this to the vendor and he was confused. I too felt confused. My friend wanted me to fight with him, but I said that it was okay.

[O/f/1,2/ii]

- Arguments.

[A/m/foll. discussion]

- Argument with a taxi-rickshaw driver who refused to stop at the right place.

[A/m/foll. discussion]

- I was having a discussion with my teacher. I put forth my point which he did not like, but ultimately after the discussion I was proved right. I felt I was right and had been let down.

[B/m/*,*/i]

- I am watching a movie. The scene is of a hill with a curved, narrow road. Suddenly there is a motorcycle falling down. At the same time, there is chaos in the auditorium, and suddenly a few terrorists appear and open fire. I ask the man next to me what has happened. He says that Mother Teresa has been killed. I feel that all the people who are devoted are not wanted in this world.

[R/m/*,*/i]

- I have gone to a friend's house with my fiancé. His family thinks that I am their future daughter-in-law. They are very excited, happy, are rejoicing and emotional. They wash my feet with milk[1], and make special food for me. I wonder how my friend can behave like this when he knows that I am going steady with someone else. But I keep quiet by telling myself that I have to do what I want and not what others want. His grandmother says she is very happy that we are getting married and that she can die in peace. She asks me to press her feet and I do it, although I always

---

[1]   Indian custom.

believed I would never touch anyone's feet. I wonder what my fiancé might think of me, whether he feels I have some real feelings towards these people. We leave when everyone is asleep. I express surprise about our friend's behaviour. My fiancé says that I should have cleared their misconception in the beginning. I say that I did not want to disappoint them as they were so happy, and that it did not make any difference to us anyway as we were to get married.

[O/f/1,1/i]

- Performance, seminars.

[A/m/foll. discussion]

- Quickly moving from one side to another, writing books.

[A/in/*,*/i]

- My exams are two months away and I am unprepared. I do not have any notes and I have to xerox some. The xerox machine is in the place that we keep an idol of a deity. I hastily move the idol and the holy books and try to xerox the notes. I am anxious, fearful and reproach myself that I have not studied.

[M/m/*,*/i]

- Known people, friends, relatives in danger.

[A/m/foll. discussion]

- Religious place, monk giving lectures.

[E/m/1,1/i]

- I am listening to my father talk about a religious lecture he had attended. Later, I fell asleep on my mother's lap.

[P/m/1,1/i]

- My friend had died; his mother was informing me of this. I had no feeling; it didn't matter. I went to play cricket.

[B/m/*,*/i]

- I was standing in a field in front of a house in a rural area. It was dark. I got the urge to pass stool. At first, I thought of going into the farm for that purpose but later I changed my mind and went towards the latrine in the house. Two girls also entered the latrine at the same time, and I gave them some clothes I had washed some time ago.

[H/m/1,1/i]

- I went to college dressed only in shorts and a vest. A girl teased me. I was embarrassed.

[F/m/1,1/i]

- A swollen scrotum with superficial ulcers on it.

[A/m/*,*]

- I am in bed with my wife and a common friend of ours. I make love with both of them.

[N/m/*,*/i]

- I was unable to attend the first day of my hospital job because I had to attend a college lecture.

[C/f/1,1/i]

- Vague, unconnected, in bits.

[E/f/1,1/i]

- Native place.

[E/f/1,1/i]

- Train journey, crowded railway station.

[E/f/1,1/i]

- I had gone an hour late to the out-patient clinic. The honorary physician sarcastically told me that henceforth he too would come an hour or so late.

[F/m/1,1/i]

- I was with an honorary physician who thought the patient before us needed *Thuja*. He asked the patient whether he had dreams of falling. When the patient was unable to confirm this, he asked whether the patient felt as if something was falling in him. I thought it was a ridiculous question and to my relief the patient answered that he did not.

[G/m/*,*/i]

- Dead mother.

[J'/m/*,*/0]

- My wife is telling me that I understand things well on the theoretical level, but on the practical level in everyday life, I behave completely different. I feel guilty because I know that she is right. I then look into the Synthetic Repertory and see the exact rubric of this symptom.

[K/m/1,2/i]

- Found myself in a dirty place in Bombay (where I had been the day before) with a beautiful view of the sea. Had a sudden insight into the cases of some patients and could come to their homoeopathic remedies.

[K/m/1,4/i]

- I am talking with my friends when suddenly the weather becomes stormy and cloudy as if it will rain. All my friends are in a very cheerful mood, and they rush to deck themselves in lovely dresses. They begin to dance in a group to drum beats. I am merely a spectator to all this.

[O/m/1,1/i]

- Going to a picnic in a bus.

[O/m/1,1/i]

- My mother was asking me about my fiancée's nature. I could feel warmth and care.

[P/m/1,1/i]

- I am searching for place to sit in a lecture. My friend, who is not supposed to take the lecture, starts to speak. He mispronounces a word and the students laugh at him. Then he says something which students repeat with wrong pronunciation. I am feeling very sleepy. The lecturer calls my name and praises me, but I cannot keep awake.

[P/m/1,2/i]

PHYSICAL SYMPTOMS

Generalities

- Tiredness in the morning.

[D/m/*,*i]

- Desire for open air.

[G/m/*,*/i]

- Chilliness.

[O/f/*,*/*]

- Better after passing stool.

[J'/m/*,*/0]

Physical particulars

Head
- Heaviness in the head, on waking in the morning, and lasting for a while afterwards.

[A/m/*,*/i]

- Heaviness in the head, not ameliorated by coffee (which is usual). Aggravated from lying down at night.

[I/m/1,3/i]

- Head pain from hunger.

[O/f/1,3/*]

Face
- Acne.

[D/m/*,*/i]

- Heat of the face, as if feeling feverish; lasted throughout the day.

[F/m/1,2/i]

Stomach
- Foul tasting eructations.
[J'/m/1,3/0]

Abdomen
- Mild indigestion with heaviness in the abdomen.
[I/m/1,1/i]
- Heaviness and uneasiness in the abdomen.
[I/m/1,3/i]

Stool
- Sudden, hard stools.
[D/m/*,*/i]
- Constant, unsatisfactory urge for stool.
[E/f/*,*/i]
- Frequency of stools with mucus. Felt that the passage of stool would ameliorate the sensation of heaviness in the abdomen.
[I/m/1,3/i]
- Frequent, urgent loose motions.
[J'/m/*,*/0]
- Constipation, straining at stool.
[J'/m/*,*/0]

Respiration
- Breathlessness after walking long. Could not sit in a closed room. Dyspnoea, accompanied by cough.
[O/f/1,3/*]
- Breathlessness in the morning.
[O/f/1,5/*]

Cough
- Cough, with dyspnoea, lasting until noon (1.30 p.m.).
[O/f/1,3/*]

Back
- Slight backache, aggravated from lying down.
[O/f/1,1/i]

- Pustular eruption on back, painful to touch.
[O/f/1,1/i]

Extremities
- Itching in the sole of the right foot.
[D/m/*,*/i]
- Pain in one spot, on medial aspect of right thigh, aggravated from touch.
[E/f/1,1/i]
- Pain in the left wrist, as if sprained, aggravated from pressure.
[F/m/1,3/i]
- Pain in the right elbow.
[F/m/1,3/i]
- Sharp, needle-like, neuralgic pain in one spot on the lateral side of the left thigh, burning, as though a hot needle was inserted in. Have to constantly check if there is something there. Worse touch, contact of clothing, walking. Troublesome pain which prevents me from walking easily.
[A/m/*,*/i]
- Intense numbness in the right thigh. Very much aggravated from touch.
[N/m/*,*/i]
- Sensation of electricity passing through leg and thigh.
[N/m/*,*/i]

Sleep
- Drowsiness all day.
[C/f/1,3/i]
- Sleepiness in the morning.
[D/m/*,*/i]
- Short sleep, but no exhaustion the following day.
[K/m/1,1/i]

Skin
- Sensation of a pin pricking in one small spot.
[J'/m/*,*/0]

RUBRICS

Mind

Single symptoms

— Anger, helpful, bystanders, at.

— Anger, understood, at, not being.

— Delusion, lost, away from this world, listening to religious songs, while.

— Ditched, feels.

— Dreams, amorous, coition with two women.

— Dreams, animals, alligators, pursued by.

— Dreams, arguments.

— Dreams, arresting deceitful cabbie.

— Dreams, angry, at injustice done to his mother.

— Dreams, bordering premises with thorny trees.

— Dreams, children, being requested to help, unescorted.

— Dreams, cycling.

— Dreams, children, shriveled up, with tear-filled eyes.

— Dreams, children, rescuing, abandoned.

— Dreams, car being filled with water.

— Dreams, cloudy weather.

— **Dreams, danger, protecting others from**.

— Dreams, dirty place with beautiful sea-view.

— Dreams, being foreigner in danger from violent persons.

— Dreams, falling asleep in his mother's lap.

— Dreams, friends, seeing, in a cheerful mood.

— Dreams, guided, being, lost, when.

— Dreams, grandmother, trying to keep a cow away from his old.

— *Dreams, helping people weaker than himself*.

— Dreams, high places, jumping off a tall building into the water.

— Dreams, hill, with curved, narrow road.

— *Dreams, injustice*.

— Dreams, kicked in the abdomen.

— Dreams, lost, guided by a policeman when lost in a strange place.

— Dreams, motorcycle, falling.

— Dreams, monk lecturing in a religious place.

— Dreams, offering his seat to a woman.

— Dreams, performance, of.

— Dreams, playing, though informed about death of friend.

— *Dreams, police*.

— Dreams, police, she must tell that her brother killed her sister.

— Dreams, political procession.

— **Dreams, protecting**.

— Dreams, protecting, wanting to protect a young boy who fell overboard.

— Dreams, protective feeling towards foreign woman.

— Dreams, playing, though informed about death of friend.

— Dreams, quickly moving from one side to another, writing books.

— Dreams, reproaching himself, for not having studied for exams.

— Dreams, riding up narrow, flooded river.
— Dreams, relatives and friends in danger.
— Dreams, rural house.
— Dreams, scrotum swollen and ulcerated.
— Dreams, striking two men who passed an obscene comments.
— Dreams, seeing her brother murder her sister.
— Dreams, slipping back into the water on attempting to drive up the steep bank of a beach.
— Dreams, terrorists, open fire in cinema hall.
— Dreams, teacher being sarcastic.
— Dreams, urge to pass stool.
— Exertion, physical, desire, vigorous, for, but walking is difficult.
— Egotism, self-esteem, others are stupid and thick, feels.
— Irritability, time wasted, about.
— Protect, desire to.
— Self-control, alternating with loss of self-control.
— Singing, midnight.
— Tranquillity, irritability, followed, by.
— Wring neck, impulse to.

Common symptoms
— *Anger, irascibility.*
— Cheerfulness, gaiety, happiness, mirth.
— Cheerfulness, evening.
— Cheerfulness, night.
— Censorious.
— Concentration difficult.
— Confusion, of mind.
— Contradict, disposition to.

— Contradiction, intolerance of.
— Delusion, animals.
— Delusion, animals, birds sees.
— Delusion, deceived.
— Delusion, neglected, he was.
— Dreams, amorous.
— Dreams, animals.
— Dreams, animals, goats.
— *Dreams, attacked, of being.*
— Dreams, danger.
— Dreams, dead relatives.
— Dreams, embarrassment.
— Dreams, fights.
— Dreams, journeys.
— Dreams, murder.
— Dreams, native country.
— Dreams, picnic.
— Dreams, pleasant.
— Dreams, quarrels.
— Dreams, religious.
— Dreams, unsuccessful efforts to do various things.
— Egotism, self-esteem.
— Forsaken feeling.
— Impatience
— Indolence.
— Irritability.
— Kill, desire to.
— Kill, desire to, knife, with a.
— Kill, desire to, sudden impulse to.
— Malicious.
— Obstinate.
— Quarrelsome.
— Rudeness.
— *Sadness, melancholy.*
— Sadness, alternating with cheerfulness.

— Sensitive, oversensitive, light, to.
— Sensitive, oversensitive, noise, to.
— Striking.
— Strike, desire to.
— Suspicious, mistrustful.
— Talk, indisposed to, desire to remain

silent, taciturn.
— Time passes too slowly.
— Tranquility, serenity, calmness.
— Unfeeling, hard-hearted.
— Weeping, tearful mood.
— Weeping, tearful mood, afternoon.

Physical symptoms

Generals
– Activity increased, afternoon, until.
– Activity, desires.
– Air open, desire for.
– Cold, aggravates.
– Lie down, desire to.
– Short sleep ameliorates.
– Weakness, morning.

Head
– Heaviness.
– Heaviness, morning.
– Heaviness, morning, waking, on.
– Heaviness, night.
– Heaviness, lying, while.
– Pain, fasting, from.

Face
– Eruptions.
– Eruptions, acne.
– Heat.

Stomach
– Eructations, foul.

Abdomen
– Heaviness, as from a load.
– Heaviness, stool, after, ameliorates.

Rectum
– Constipation.
– Diarrhoea.
– Pain, tenesmus, stool, during.

– Urging, constant.
– Urging, sudden.

Stool
– Hard.
– Mucous.

Respiration
– Difficult.
– Difficult, morning.
– Difficult, air, open, ameliorates.
– Difficult, walking.

Cough
– Noon, until.

Back
– Eruptions, painful.
– Eruptions, pustules.
– Pain, lying, while.

Extremities
– Itching.
– Itching, lower limbs.
– Itching, lower limbs, foot, side of.
– Numbness, lower limbs, thigh, right.
– Pain, lower limbs, neuralgic.
– Pain, lower limbs, thigh, left.
– Pain, lower limbs, thigh, spot, in single.
– Pain, upper limbs, elbow.
– Pain, upper limbs, wrist.

- Pain, sprained, as if, wrist, in.
- Pain, burning, thigh, spot, in.
- Pain, lower limbs, thigh, right.
- Pain, burning, thigh, hot needles, as from.
- Pain, burning, thigh, touch aggravates.

Sleep
- Sleepiness.
- Sleepiness, daytime.
- Sleepiness, morning

Skin
- Prickling, small spot, in.

THEMES

1. Need to fight for others.

2. Attack and defence.

3. Need to protect others from attack, danger, antisocial elements. The need to police.

4. Anger at injustice.

5. Anger at not being understood.

6. Egotism: others are "thick" and stupid, and impatience from the same feeling.

7. Violent impulses. Desire to hit, to kill with a knife, to wring someone's neck.

8. Performance; anxiety before performance.

9. Unsuccessful efforts.

10. A sense of duty. Helping those weaker than himself.

11. Quarrelsomeness and malice.

12. Lonely, forsaken feeling.

13. Disposition to contradict and intolerance of contradiction.

9

THE PROVING OF *OCIMUM SANCTUM* (BASIL)

I conducted a proving of *Ocimum sanctum* with ten provers, in September 1994. The provers were each given one dose in the 30 C potency. All of them took the dose. Neither the provers nor I knew what substance was being proved. The provers noted their symptoms and met with me individually once every week over the next three weeks to report their symptoms. Prover A required a second dose of the substance before the onset of symptoms.

The drug was obtained from the pharmacy, "Roy and Company", Bombay.

MIND

Emotions

Irritability / Anger

- Feel angry towards a friend who neglected and betrayed me. Was short tempered and "to the point" when talking with him. I hadn't expected this from him; he was the only person on whom I could rely. Have lost faith in everybody, in humanity. I feel such relationships are to satisfy your ego, your need to talk, but if that person neglects you, what is the use?

[C/f/1,*/i]

- Was really "wild" at a friend for not showing up. I felt she thinks of me as "nothing", that she doesn't value me and feels she can use me as she wants. I felt I was not being given much importance, felt neglected, and was restless and nervous. She had lied to me and I was very angry and quarrelled with her, saying if this was how things were. I didn't need anyone. I wouldn't listen to any explanations.

[F/m/1,*/i]

- Irritable at trifles, following a misunderstanding with my best friend.

[I/f/1,*/i]

- Irritable on waking in the morning, ameliorated by afternoon. Was singing again in the afternoon (as she had been on the previous day).

[G/f/1,2/i]

- I was very angry with a nurse who would not allow me to attend an operation. Wanted to tell her something, but was unable to. Wanted someone to slap her and throw her out of the hospital. Felt insulted. Later complained against her, but was unable to confront her which I regretted.

[G/m/1,*/i]

Neglected / Alone

- Ego hurt from some suggestion my best friend had made; I felt that she was talking "rubbish", and that everyone was trying to break my ego. I had a feeling that someone would come up to me and tell me that I was useless. I felt like I was standing on a stage and everyone, including her, was laughing at me. I told her that I didn't want her company. I felt neglected by her; she was my best friend, yet she didn't understand me. I refused to talk to her for long, and felt that she should apologize.

[I/m/1,*/i]

- Weeping, when alone, when a very close friend ignored me. Felt he had neglected me, was avoiding me, was indifferent towards me. I hadn't expected this from him; he was the person to whom I was very close.

I felt he had betrayed me, let me down. I felt a bit insulted, that he was not treating me like a human being. I stopped talking to him for two or three days, with the feeling that I did not want to be the one to submit always. But finally I went and spoke to him, and constantly pestered him as to why he was avoiding and neglecting me. Wanted to commit suicide by taking potassium cyanide and I jokingly said to him that I would murder him before doing it.

[C/f/1,∗/i]

- Lonely feeling, as if there was no one with me when my friends attended a lecture without informing me. Felt bad that they did not inform me while I help them whenever I can. Feeling that there is no real friend here.

[H/m/1,∗/i]

Friends / Company

- Felt that my group (of nearly twenty-five people) was breaking up, and each one was doing what he wanted; felt bad as a result.

[I/m/1,∗/i]

- Nervous, tense, restless, following misunderstanding with friend. Wanted company, someone to talk to, which ameliorated.

[F/m/1,4/i]

- Tense, following misunderstanding with a friend.

[I/m/1,2/i]

- Feel better from talking to someone.

[C/f/1,∗/i]

Emotions / No emotions

- Either very emotional, or no emotions at all. When a relative passed away I was the only one who didn't weep. On the other hand, on two or three occasions, I wept for trivial matters.

[C/f/1,∗/i]

- Could enjoy myself with my other friends, but weeping when alone, feeling betrayed and neglected by my very close friend. Unusually, not brooding, nothing affects me much except this guy. Have become cold-blooded. Was unusually unaffected when a friend who was supposed to meet me didn't show up.

Have become cold-blooded, indifferent towards him (close friend) also, though I still feel he is a part of me. I think I have learnt to accept things in my life and to compromise with people and circumstances; I let things go on the way there are going.

[C/f/1,∗/i]

- Was angry, restless, and nervous, when a friend neglected me. But was unafffected the next day, and went through it laughing, singing, happy, joking with my other friends. Later, I called her to settle things but ended up blaming her. The next day, felt guilty for my behaviour and decided to forgive and forget, and felt that I should understand her problem.

[F/m/1,∗/i]

Indifference

- Indifferent; not bothered by anything. Equally unaffected by compliments, rude behaviour or insults. Felt that I had been expecting too much, and now I don't expect anything. Had no feelings at all, no emotions, no pleasure, was unable to enjoy things that used to be fun and thrilling for me. I don't think about any situation or incident anymore. It is as if my brain has stopped working.

[C/f/2,∗/i]

- Usual tension was absent when I heard exams being declared.

[G/f/1,4/i]

- Was unusually careless about dressing.

[I/m/1,2/i]

Fear / Anxiety

- Constant feeling, while riding my motorcycle that something was going to happen, although I was driving carefully. Palpitations, with the feeling that I was not going to survive, when I realized (when driving in the rain) that if my front wheel went into a pit, I would fall.

[F/m/1,3/i]

- Tremendous fear as to what will happen, since frightful dream. Fear even when the phone rings.

[I/m/1,∗/i]

- Sudden fear of accident, death. While sitting on the last seat of a bus; got up involuntarily at the thought of the possibility of an accident. Jerked fearfully on hearing a car honk behind me: it was ten feet away but a current of fear passed through me; a fear of accident or death. Intense fear of accident while sitting in a fast car, although I knew the driver to be cautious. Also, was more cautious while crossing the road.

[J/m/1,*/i]

• Palpitation and anxiety from suspense, because I was expecting a surprise from my friend the next day. Ameliorated from lying with the head propped up.

[J/m/1,6/i]

Singing

• Felt active and light in the morning. A couple of songs came to mind: "I have written my first love letter..." and "I haven't slept nor woken since ages, one day you will come...". I felt the need of a person very close to me, like a partner whom I could tell everything to.

[D/f/1,2/i]

• Woke up unusually early in the morning, lively, energetic, in an unusually happy mood, singing songs like "Our dreams are now of one colour. We will always be together..." and "My love, I look for you everywhere, we're still apart...".

[G/f/1,1/i]

• Singing – didn't want to pay attention to the lecture I was attending.

[G/f/1,2/i]

• Have been singing the song "I have to make this love grow, slowly".

[G/f/1,2/i]

• Singing in the evening with the feeling that life is full of fun and should be enjoyed to the fullest.

[G/f/1,4/i]

Miscellaneous

• Guilty that I wasn't following instructions for the proving very strictly.

[E/m/1,1/i]

• Happy with the feeling that I was getting more attention from my colleagues.

[F/m/1,2/i]

• Sense of responsibility increased. Was more mature.

[C/f/1,*/i]

• Became fond of wearing good jewellery.

[C/f/1,*/i]

• Overconfident about exams, even though had been unable to concentrate.

[J/m/1,*/i]

• Laughing involuntarily, immoderately, uncontrollably, from remembering something I had found funny two days ago.

[G/f/1,*/i]

• Odd behaviour (which had been in control all these years). For example: I would unnecessarily trouble my grandmother and if she said anything wrong I would shout. Would pick quarrels, which I have not been doing all these days.

[E/m/2,*/i]

• Told my sister about a girl I saw that she had the most beautiful eyelashes I had seen (unusual for me, I don't usually discuss such things with my sister). Felt awkward. Later, said that they are better than mine at least.

[E/m/before dose]

• Strange questions came to my mind, for example: "Can a monkey get drunk?" and "Is the man so demented?"

[E/m/1,*/i]

• Agreeably attended a religious function which I would have usually been reluctant to do. Felt pleasant, happy and emotional.

[F/m/1,*/i]

• After listening to friends' problems, felt that the same thing would happen to me.

[I/m/1,2/i]

• I volunteered, to everyone's surprise,

to give a friend some money that she had lost, saying that she didn't have to return it to me.

[G/f/1,2/i]

■ Felt sympathetic and caring towards an old aunt and agreed to spend the time with her that I usually like to spend only with my friends.

[J/m/1,1/i]

■ Capricious.

[I/m/1,*/i]

■ Indolence, sluggishness, aversion to work and study.

[I/m/1,*/i]

■ Was unable to concentrate; wanted to run away from any kind of responsibility, wanted to be free of all burdens.

[J/m/1,*/i]

Intellect

■ Dullness in the morning, lasting until midday. Felt everything was moving slow, as if nothing was going very fast. Felt that my brain was so packed up that there was no further thinking.

[D/f/1,1/i]

■ Dullness of mind.

[G/f/1,1/i]

■ Lost my way, two or three times, in a place I was quite familiar with. Had to come back to my house and take a road I was very

familiar with, before I finally got to my destination.

[E/m/1,3/i]

■ Confusion of mind, things seen seemed familiar – as if déjà vu.

[E/m/2,*/i]

■ Forgetful about whom I had lent my book to; couldn't remember even though I tried hard. Also made many spelling mistakes.

[J/m/1,4/i]

DREAMS

Anxious / Fearful

■ I was leaving my neighbour's house, was trying to shut the door but it wouldn't shut. I then noticed a strange man going to the first floor. I realized that the person on the first floor had received a death threat and I felt this was the person who had threatened him. I then saw a gun protruding out from the door that wouldn't shut. I felt fear and a tension that something would happen, that this person would kill the man on the first floor or that I would be murdered.

[B/f/1,*/i]

■ Something huge suddenly appeared when I was walking with my friends. I was

tense as to what would happen and felt it would surely destroy my friends, my village and me. I had a feeling that when the evil thing would happen, everyone would run here and there, and I would be alone with my tremendous fear about what would happen. I felt that whatever was happening was because of my bad deeds.

Then, suddenly, I felt that there was another, stronger power that was capable of destroying that evil thing and saving me. I felt a sense of hopelessness, like I couldn't do anything. I had to just leave everything to God; he would help me and everything would be okay.

A tremendous fear since that day as to what will happen.

[I/m/1,2/i]

- Pursued by murders from whom I was trying to escape. Fear of being murdered. Was telling everyone to run, otherwise they would killed. I felt I had to escape somehow in order to survive.

[G/f/1,2/i]

- My sister had fainted in college, and was brought home by a maid. She had a chit with the name of a medicine on it. I went to the chemist to buy it and was told that these medicines are used for heart block or arterial block; he advised an electrocardiogram be done. I got very scared.

[A/f/2,∗/ii]

- I was having my case taken, during which I narrated three dreams. One of them was that my mother was very angry with me and said that she will die. I got very scared, fell at her feet and wept profusely, saying that she couldn't leave me, I would miss her very much, and that I couldn't live without her or even imagine my life without her.

[G/f/1,5/i]

- Anxious and worried while waiting for exam results, till I got the news that everyone had passed, which made me happy.

[G/f/1,∗/i]

- I have failed an exam by just half a mark. I don't know how to tell my father who has accompanied me. I can't express myself, can't show him what I feel whether I am happy or sad. Everyone around me is happy, and I don't know what I should tell my father. Woke up frightened.

[A/f/2,∗/ii]

Danger

- I was riding on a motorcycle with a friend, when we halted at a railway crossing. My cousins were in a car next to me; they were going to my house. As the gate opened, I started my bike and went through only to find another gate. There were seven to eight such gates, one after the other, opening and closing alternately. There was some old machinery around me, but no roads. One of my cousins who had been in the car came alone on a motorcycle and he, too, was surprised at all this. He asked me what was to be done and I replied that I did not know. I felt that this is a trap for me from which I couldn't get out, and felt that I would die there.

[F/m/1,1/i]

- I was very poor, had no money, and was living in a hut with my family. A friend, along with her doctor husband came to stay with us. Her husband got called to see a very sick child.

Suddenly, I looked out of the window and noticed that there was sea all around. I was a bit shaky on looking out, scared as to how the house was on water, and that if it fell into the water, we would all drown.

There was also an old woman in the house who was constantly talking, irritating and harassing others.

[G/f/1,∗/i]

- I see a truck run over a man. I run over to his side immediately thinking that he must have fractured a lot of ribs, and that perhaps I could see a case of flail chest with all its classical signs. But as I approach, the scene changes.

The place now is narrow and there is a huge truck heavily loaded with some metal covered with tarpaulin or canvas. The metal is not balanced properly, and starts to fall on us. There are people, both in front of me and behind me. Everyone turns around, and the man in front of me is moving slowly. I want him to move fast, I feel I will get crushed now. I don't tell him anything, but there is a sense of urgency to get out of the place.

[E/m/2,∗/i]

Anger and violence

- My aunt wanted her nails painted.

I agreed to do it for her, but she refused, saying that I didn't know how to and that I would spoil them. I felt she had insulted me in front of all her friends. I was angry, and felt she should have been polite.

[G/f/1,2/i]

- My mother was getting me married to an ugly, weird-looking fellow with some skin disease. I was not aware about the marriage or how it was happening. I was very angry with my mother, feeling it was nonsense, and how could she get me married to someone so dirty! I found him very filthy, and woke up relieved that it was a dream.

[A/f//2,*/ii]

- I am transcribing some notes. My father does not seem to like this and shows some displeasure on his face. I feel tense, as if he would shout at someone or that there might be a fight if I don't stop. I continue to work with tension and discomfort, all the time worried that there could be a fight. I feel angry and oppressed; I feel I am not doing anything wrong but if there is a fight, I will be responsible for it. At one point, I can't bear it anymore. Something snaps in me, and I go to his room, wait for him to say something and start to beat him up very badly. I feel for no fault of mine he is angry and I will do the same to him.

[E/m/1,1/i]

- Injustice, being cheated and violently fighting back.

[E/m/1,1/i]

- My friend is being beaten very badly by one of his teachers. I don't know why she is doing it – he is a good student, never mischievous. I ask her why, and she starts to beat me instead. I get very angry; she is beating me unnecessarily. I take the scale from her hand and start to beat her.

[H/m/1,*/i]

Friends

- I was in a train with my friends. We were all playing cards. I was to get off at a particular station along with a friend of mine. Suddenly, I realized that the train had long past my station. I told my friend, who was to alight with me, but she said she was going to another friends place and would get off elsewhere. I felt angry, ditched, cheated and insulted by her and felt that she should have informed me. I got off three stations ahead with my luggage to board another train. All the compartments of this train were of the first class. The guard saw that I was trying to catch the train, but the train started. I felt he had ditched me, and felt helpless.

Later, on reaching home, I found one of my bags missing. I couldn't remember where I had it with me or not. Suddenly, I found it under my cupboard, and did not know how it got there.

[B/f/2,*/i]

- My friend had borrowed the "Organon of Medicine" from the college library and not returned it for long. I needed the same book and kept requesting him to lend it to me. He kept postponing it. I got very angry, wanted to do something to teach him a lesson. I felt whenever he asked me for something, I gave it to him readily, and he had been refusing me. I took the book from his bag without his knowledge. When he found out and questioned me, I was high-tempered, and said: "Whenever you ask me for something I give it readily, and you have been refusing me this book though I have asked you for so long."

Woke up with palpitations and perspiration. Couldn't go back to sleep.

[H/m/1,*/i]

- I visited the shop of a friend. I liked a white purse with many small mirrors. My friend told me it cost five hundred rupees. I thought it was very costly.

[B,f/1,*/i]

- Friends – pleasant

[B/f/1,*/i]

Amazement / Surprise

- I was roaming in a big institution when I got the news that my mother's friend had died. I went outside of a room, and through the windows I could see some people chanting mantras. A watchman, standing beside me, pointed that behind me was the body of the dead woman. There was a foul odour and I moved back. I also saw four or five dead infants and was told they died in labour as did their mother. I was confused as my friend's mother had been a widow [1]. I was amazed, unable to understand the situation, was trying to catch up with it, but was unable to. The pace of things was very fast.

[F/m/1,1/i]

- My aunt had two pets: a small white dog and a housefly. I was very surprised as to how she could keep a housefly as a pet. I asked her how she was able to differentiate her housefly from all others around. She said she was able to recognize it. Whenever I went, her pets would follow me around – the dog at my feet and the housefly at my head. I asked her: "Why do you keep such silly pets in the house?"

[A/f/2,*/ii]

Alone

- I was waiting for someone or something when a big vehicle appeared. I entered it, and just as the doors were about to close I saw three-four big men attacking me. I could see their big hands coming towards me, and I got very scared. I screamed for help. I had the feeling that one of my classmates was outside, and I called out to him. But there seemed to be nobody there. I had the feeling that no one was going to come and help me, I can't depend on anyone. Whatever I have to do I should do it on my own. I have to fight for myself. So I just pushed those people

---

[1] Very unusual in Indian Society for an unmarried or widowed woman to have sexual relations.

and ran out.

[A/f/1,*/ii]

- Was on a picnic with my relatives. The place, though new, seemed familiar; in fact, I was showing my cousin around. We had to cross a stream of water when I suddenly realized that I was alone on one side of it. I was looking around for people – where could they have gone? I felt all alone. Then a cousin came searching for me saying that everyone was waiting for me to join them for lunch.

[D/f/1,*/i]

- My mother was pregnant, I felt awkward. I assumed I would have a baby brother. I remembered my sister's friend who had delivered a baby girl two years ago, and had felt awkward and embarrassed about it. I also remembered a classmate whose sister was very much older than her and she felt lonely and distanced from her. I decided that I would not let my brother feel lonely.

[E/m/1,*/i]

Miscellaneous

- There were many interns posted in the usually empty Out-Patient Clinic that I attend. The honorary physician was teaching. I felt good that so many people were attending (usually I feel that he teaches well and no one attends).

[B/f/1,*/i]

- Was in charge of a ship, along with a friend, and we had to catch smugglers. We did catch them and I was very happy about it. (Had been reading a book with similar contents.)

[B/f/2,*/i]

- There is a lot of commotion around. I am told that there was a fire in which a lot of people had died. I start running towards the spot, not so much to help them but to see what is happening, for the sake of curiosity. I have to cross a public garden which is closed for the day, but I run through it nonetheless. The gardener is sitting there and I have the feeling that he will stop me, but he does not. It starts to rain, my clothes get wet and I feel that it is a nuisance. I reach the place, everything is black, scorched and burnt and the police are there to control the crowd. As I move closer to have a look, a policeman pushes me away but then, recognizing me as the nephew of an important police official, goes away without saying anything. I look at the place: there is a temple with a few people sitting inside but not much chaos to suggest that there had been a fire. I feel my curiosity has been satisfied. Also as I approach the place, my wet clothes start to dry up, and I feel very happy about it.

[E/m/2,∗/i]

- I saw an accident where three trains had dashed against each other to form a pattern like an arrow; no feeling.

[F/m/1,5/i]

- I am at a marriage where I have eaten too much. I bend to pick up something, and I vomit so much that I faint.

[A/f/2,∗/ii]

- I was eating lunch with my family, there were many tasty food items. But I had to control myself because I was on a diet. Felt that I couldn't eat what I wanted to.

[G/f/1,5/i]

- We had to prove a remedy prepared from the mouse. Saw a cat chase a mouse.

[B/f/1,∗/i]

- I have to be in the hospital at 9.30 a.m. but for some reason am unable to go. Later, I think that I should still try and make it. I looked at my watch, it was 11.30 a.m., but I am still not able to go. Again I think I should go and when I check the time in my watch, it is 1.30 p.m. I feel that I should still go. I feel helpless for some reason and am finally unable to go.

[B/f/2,∗/i]

- Pleasant dream of being on a picnic.

[B/f/1,∗/i]

- Cousin.

[D/f/i,∗/i]

- I have gone into a secret room, taken a book and come out into another room. My sister enters and I do not want her to see the book because then she will know I have been to the secret room. I try desperately to distract her. She is almost going to find out, when I show her some jars of food that my mother has prepared. All of them are stale except the last one which contains some good food, and with which she gets distracted and leaves.

[E/m/1,1/i]

- I was at an opera with my sister. She was showing me some semi-nude pictures of famous film actress from a thick book. There was a feeling of openness. But when my sister looked away, I tried to peep into the book again, and felt guilty about this.

[E/m/1,1/i]

- Reading a textbook and marking in it with a highlighter.

[E/m/1,4/i]

- I was dressed up to go out somewhere, and waiting for someone. I felt happy and excited. Then for some reason, I was upset and all the excitement was gone.

[G/f/1,1/i]

- I have dressed up for my aunt's wedding when my grandmother says she will give me a better dress. She opens a cupboard and from it she gives me a beautiful dress. I am happy. Then I notice that she is breathless. I tell her not to give me the dress, and say that it is okay if I don't have it, and that she is more important than the dress. I return it to her saying I will take her to a doctor.

[G/f/∗,∗/i]

- A person got into a small box and disappeared.

[J/m/1,2/i]

- Talking to a neighbour who had returned from Dubai.

[J/m/1,2/i]

- My uncles were playing with marbles and were quarrelling for single pieces.
[J/m/1,3/i]

PHYSICAL SYMPTOMS

Generalities

- Desire for chilled lemon juice, spicy food and snacks, sandwiches.
[B/f/1,*/i]
- Desire for snacks, pizza.
[C/f/1,*/i]
- Desires juicy things, cold drinks, ice lollies.
[D/f/1,*/i]
- Thirst increased.
[G/f/1,*/i]
- Desires pineapple juice, juicy things, cold drinks.
[G/f/1,*/i]
- Increased thirst for cool water.
[J/m/1,2/i]

- Bone pains throughout the day.
[D/f/1,*/i]
- Feeling hot with perspiration.
[D/f/1,*/i]
- Tiredness through the day.
[D/f/1,*/i]
- Fainting from hunger.
[F/m/1,4/i]
- Extreme fatigue, weakness, feverish feeling in the afternoon.
[G/f/1,5/i]
- Not tired despite exertion throughout the day.
[G/f/1,*/i]

Physical particulars

Head
- Headache in the morning.
[A/f/1,*/ii]
- Pain in right temple on opening the mouth.
[B/f/1,*/i]
- Generalized throbbing headache from hunger.
[C/f/1,*/i]
- Heaviness in the head with coryza.
[C/f/1,*/i]
- Occipital headache and profuse sweat on forehead during fainting attack.
[F/m/1,4/i]
- Throbbing headache in the evening from over-exertion and hunger, with visible carotid pulsation.
[J/m/1,3/i]
- Severe headache in temples as if compressing the brain, with a stretching sensation extending to the cheeks. Aggravated around 12.30 - 1.00 a.m., midnight, and ameliorated in the morning. Tossing about with the pain.
[C/f/2,* i]

- Head pain: frontal, occipital, over the eyes. Ameliorated from pressure, and from boring the head into a pillow. Aggravated between 9.00 p.m. and 11.00 p.m.

[J/m/before dose]

Eye

- Lachrymation in the morning.

[A/f/1,*/ii]

- Swelling, both eyelids with, sticky discharge.

[J/m/before dose]

Ear

- Fullness in ears, during fainting attack.

[F/m/1,*/i]

- Small boil in left ear.

[F/m/1,*/i]

Nose

- A lot of sneezing in the morning.

[A/f/1,*/ii]

- Sneezing, aggravated on waking up in the morning. Eight to nine sneezes at a time. Aggravated from cold lemonade.

[B/f/1,*/i]

- Nose block.

[B/f/1,*/i]

- Coryza, with heaviness in the head.

[C/f/1,*/i]

- Continuous sneezing, ten to twelve sneezes at a time, aggravated on waking in the morning.

[E/f/1,*/i]

- Coryza, on waking in the morning, upto 12.00 noon. Ameliorated after eating.

[J/m/1,*/i]

- Severe left-sided nose block, with headache.

[C/f/1,*/i]

- Sneezing from getting the feet wet.

[J/m/1,*/i]

Mouth

- Painful aphtous ulcers on the upper

lip, between the two incisors. Lasted one month.

[E/m/1,*/i]

- Dryness in mouth with increased thirst.

[J/m/1,2/i]

- Bad taste in mouth, worse after waking.

[J/m/1,2/i]

Throat

- Pain in the throat .

[G/f/*,*/i]

- Itching, burning in the oesophagus, ameliorated drinking cold water.

[H/m/1,*/i]

Stomach

- Appetite increased. Hungry five minutes after eating, but don't eat much. Easy satiety.

[C/f/1,*/i]

- Thirst increased.

[G/f/1,*/i]

- Stomach pain, better from bending.

[H/m/1,*/i]

Abdomen

- Pain just below the umbilicus, as if a thread is pulling it backwards. Aggravated on bending backwards, ameliorated from passing stool.

[E/m/1,*/i]

- Fullness in the abdomen, lasting long after stool.

[E/m/1,*/i]

Stool

- Soft stool with much straining.

[E/m/1,*/i]

- Constipation every alternate day, with peculiar odour in stool.

[I/m/1,*/i]

- White-coloured worm in stool.

[J/m/*,*/i]

Bladder

- Increased frequency of urination.
  [E/m/1,*/i]
- Frequent irritation.
  [I/m/1,*/i]

Urine

- White, milky, turbid in the morning.
  [J/m/*,*/i]

Male

- Itching in groins at night.
  [F/m/1,*/i]

Cough

- Cough with pain in the chest. Aggravated from yawning, from deep inspiration. Initially dry cough, then productive.
  [B/f/1,*/i]

Expectoration

- Creamish-coloured, sweetish-tasting expectoration, sometimes easy to bring up, but mostly difficult.
  [B/f/1,*/i]

Chest

- Pain in the ribs.
  [D/f/1,*/i]
- Palpitations, anxiety and sleeplessness in anticipation of a surprise.
  [J/ /*,*/i]
- Very small eruption on the right side of the chest, of reddish brown colour with black dots, and with rough surface.
  [C/f/*,*/i]
- Pain at one point of the sternum. Aggravated from coughing, yawning.
  [B/f/1,*/i]

Back

- Itching.
  [F/m/1,2,i]
- Back pain in the afternoon .
  [F/m/1,2/i]

Extremities

- Left knee pain at night.
  [A/f/1,*/ii]
- Pain in the right leg without having exerted myself at all.
  [D/f/1,*/i] (D)
- Itching on thighs in the evening.
  [F/m/1,2/i]
- Sudden, severe, intolerable, pain in the right knee lasting the whole day. Aggravated from flexing the knee, sitting, climbing stairs, pressure, cold. Ameliorated from touch, hot water application.
  [G/f/1,*/i]

Sleep

- Feeling drowsy, yawning a lot.
  [B/f/1,*/i]
- Jerking of the whole body during sleep, sudden. Awoke with a jerk.
  [C/f/1,*/i]
- Sleeplessness till 1.00 - 1.30 a.m. Then waking late between 9.00 and 9.15 a.m.
  [C/f/1,*/i]
- Sleeplessness till 1.00 -2.00 a.m. Then awake all night.
  [C/f/2,*/i]
- Yawning throughout the day, despite having slept well.
  [D/f/1,*/i]
- Waking up unrefreshed in the morning.
  [E/m/1,*/i]
- Waking up earlier than usual, feeling lively and energetic.
  [G/f/1,1/i
- Drowsiness.
  [G/f/1,5/i]
- Sleepy at 4.00 - 5.00 p.m.
  [J/m/1,5/i]
- Sleeplessness with anxiety and palpitations in anticipation of a surprise. Couldn't

lie flat. Had to lie propped up.

[J/m/1,4/i]

▪ Sleepy in the mornings. Tremendous unrefreshed feeling. Feel like closing my eyes when at work.

[E/m/2,∗/i]

Fever

▪ Mild fever with slight bodyache.

[B/f/1,∗/i]

▪ High fever with weakness.

[H/f/1,∗/i]

RUBRICS

Mind

Single symptoms

— Anxiety, lying with head raised ameliorates.

— Delusion, afflicted, he would be, with the same problems that were bothering his friends.

— Delusion, ego, everyone was trying to hurt her.

— Dreams, accidents, collision of three trains.

—– Dreams, alone, against a huge, destructive force.

— Dreams, amazement that widow had given birth.

— Dreams, animals, insects, housefly, aunt had a pet.

— Dreams, attacked by big men.

— Dreams, beaten, teacher, by.

— Dreams, beating, father, his.

— Dreams, cheated, he was being.

— Dreams, danger, murder, of.

— Dreams, danger, trapped, of being.

— Dreams, dead infants.

— Dreams, diet.

— Dreams, ditched, she had been.

— Dreams, dressing for a wedding.

— Dreams, embarrassment, his mother was pregnant.

— Dreams, fear, sister will discover his secret room.

— Dreams, fights, fight for herself, she had to, there being no one to depend upon.

— Dreams, fights, fighting back violently, injustice, against.

— Dreams, fire, burned and scorched, everything had been.

— Dreams, friends, cheated by.

— Dreams, friends, ditched by.

— Dreams, frightened, of being, to find out that her sister had a heart disease.

— Dreams, gates, opening and shutting in succession.

— Dreams, malicious, of being, towards friend who had refused him help.

— Dreams, marriage, forced to marry an ugly man with a skin disease.

— Dreams, narrow place.

— Dreams, oppressed, being.

— Dreams, people, person disappearing into a small box.

— Dreams, pictures, sister was showing him, semi-nude.

— Dreams, poor, she was.

— Dreams, pursued, murderers, by.

— Dreams, relatives, grandmother, sick, she had to rush to the doctor.

— Dreams, separated, relatives, from.

— Dreams, truck, heavily loaded, tilting towards them.

— Dreams, water, house was on.

— Dreams, weeping profusely at the idea that her mother would die.

— Dreams, woman, old, irritating and harrassing others.

— Dullness, morning, noon, until.

— Jewellery, desires to wear.

— *Quarrelsomeness, scolding, friends, with.*

— *Singing, romantic songs.*

— Suicidal disposition, poisoning by cyanide.

Common symptoms
- Activity, morning.
- **Ailments from disappointment, deception.**
- Ailments from indignation.
- Ailments from love, disappointed.
- Ailments from mortification, chagrin.
- Anxiety, palpitations, with.
- Capricious.
- Cautious.
- Company, desire for.
- Concentration, difficult.
- Confusion of mind, loses his way in well-known streets.
- Conscientious, trifles, about.
- Conversation ameliorates.
- Delusion, experienced before, thought, everything had been.
- Delusion, friendless.
- Delusion, injury, will receive.
- Delusion, insulted, he or she is.
- Delusion, laughed at, mocked, being.
- Delusion, neglected, she is.
- Dreams, accidents.
- Dreams, animals, cat pursuing a mouse (*Coca-Cola*).
- Dreams, anxious.
- Dreams, danger.
- Dreams, danger, death, of.
- Dreams, danger, drowning, of.
- Dreams, dead bodies.
- Dreams, embarrassment.
- Dreams, evil, impending.
- Dreams, friends.
- Dreams, frightful.
- Dreams, frightful, fear, followed by.
- Dreams, guns.
- Dreams, picnics.
- Dreams, pleasant.
- Dreams, pursued.
- Dreams, quarrels.
- Dreams, rain, of being soaked in.
- Dreams, relatives.
- Dreams, running.
- Dreams, weddings.
- Dullness, sluggishness, difficulty in thinking.
- Fear, accidents.
- Fear, crossing streets.
- Fear, death, of.
- Fear, falling, of.
- *Fear, happen, something will.*
- Forgetfulness.
- Forsaken feeling.
- Indifference.
- Indolence, aversion to work.
- Irritability, morning, waking, on.
- Irritability, noon ameliorates.
- Irritability trifles, at.
- Laughing, involuntary.
- Laughing, uncontrollable.
- Malicious.
- Mistakes makes, spelling, in.
- Religious affections.
- Senses, dullness, of blunted.
- *Singing.*
- Singing, morning.
- Singing, evening.
- Sympathetic.
- Talk, desires to, to someone.
- Torments others.
- Weeping, tearful mood, alone, when.
- Weeping, tearful mood, easily.

Physical symptoms

Generalities
- Faintness, hunger, from.
- Food and drink, cold drink, cold water, desires.
- Food and drink, ice, desires.
- Food and drink, juicy things, desires.
- Food and drink, lemonade, aggravates.
- Food and drink, lemonade, desires.
- Food and drink, pinepapple, desires, juice (single).
- Food and drink, spices, desires.
- Heat, sensation of.
- Jerking, sleep, during.
- Pain, bones, of.
- Weakness.
- Weakness, daytime.
- Weakness, afternoon.
- Weariness.

Head
- Heaviness.
- *Pain.*
- Pain, morning.
- Pain, morning, 9.00 a.m. - 11.00 a.m. (single).
- Pain, accompanied by, nose, obstruction of.
- Pain, boring head into pillow, ameliorates (single).
- Pain, pressure, external, ameliorates.
- Pain, forehead.
- Pain, forehead, eyes, above.
- Pain, occiput.
- Pain, temples, opening mouth.
- Pain, pressing, morning, ameliorates.
- Pain, pressing, noon.
- Pain, pressing, afternoon.
- Pain, pressing, brain.
- Pain, pressing, temples.
- Perspiration, forehead.
- Pulsating.
- Pulsating, evening.
- Pulsating, hunger from (single).
- Pulsating, temples, vessels.

Eye
- Discharges, viscid.
- Lachrymation, morning.
- Swelling, lids.

Ear
- Eruptions, boils, left (single).
- Fullness, sensation of.

Nose
- Coryza.
- Coryza, morning, waking.
- Coryza, noon, until (single).
- Coryza, eating ameliorates (single).
- *Sneezing.*
- Sneezing, morning.
- Sneezing, morning, waking, on.
- Sneezing, constant.
- Sneezing, paroxysmal.
- Sneezing, wet feet, from getting.
- Obstruction.

Mouth
- Aphtae.
- Aphtae, gums, incisors between (single).
- Aphtae, lip, upper, inside of (single).
- Dryness, thirst, with.
- Taste, bad, morning, waking, on.

Throat
- Itching.
- Pain.
- Pain, burning.
- Pain, burning, drinks, cold ameliorate.

Stomach
- Appetite, easy satiety.
- Appetite, increased.
- Appetite, ravenous, eating, after eating, soon.
- Pain, bending ameliorates (single).
- Thirst.

Abdomen
- Fullness, sensation of.
- Pain, drawing, umbilicus.
- Pain, drawing, umbilicus, bending backwards (single).
- Pain, drawing, umbilicus, stool, after, ameliorates (single).
- Pain, drawing, umbilicus, extending to back (single).

Rectum
- Constipation.
- Constipation, difficult stool, soft stool.
- Worms, complaints of worms.

Stool
- Soft.

Bladder
- Urination, frequent.

Urine
- Cloudy, morning.
- Milky, morning.
- Sediment, white.

Male
- Itching, night.
- Itching, thighs, between.

Cough
- Breathing, deep.
- Dry.
- Yawning.

Expectoration
- Cream-like, yellowish white.
- Difficult.
- Taste, sweetish.

Chest
- Eruptions, red.
- Eruptions, side, right (single).
- Pain, cough, during.
- Pain, small spots.
- Pain, yawning.
- Pain, ribs.
- Palpitations, anxiety, with.

Back
- Itching.
- Pain, afternoon.

Extremities
- Itching, thigh, evening.
- Pain, knee.
- Pain, knee, right.
- Pain, knee, left.
- Pain, knee, ascending stairs, on.
- Pain, knee, flexing limb.
- Pain, knee, pressure aggravates.
- Pain, knee, sitting, while.
- Pain, knee, touch, on.
- Pain, knee, warmth ameliorates.

Sleep
- Sleepiness.
- Sleepiness, morning. waking, on.
- Sleepiness, afternoon, 4.00 p.m. - 5.00 p.m. (single).
- Sleepiness, eyes, opening difficult.

- Sleepiness, work, during.
- Sleeplessness.
- Sleeplessness, midnight, after, 1.00 a.m. or 2.00 a.m., until.
- Sleeplessness, anxiety, from.
- Sleeplessness, excitement, from.

- Sleeplessness, palpitation, from.
- Unrefreshing.
- Waking, jerks, by.
- Yawning.
- Yawning, daytime.

THEMES

1. Being let down, betrayed, neglected, cheated by her best friend or the person she felt closest to.

2. Being ditched by the person she depended or relied on.

3. Feeling that her friends did not value her, that they were using her.

4. Feeling alone and friendless that all his friends deserted him.

5. Feeling insulted.

6. Feeling laughed at.

7. Feeling that those close to her did not understand her.

8. Being unaffected by everything else except the behaviour of the person she felt closest to.

9. Tormenting and pestering her best friend for having let her down.

10. Amelioration from company, from conversation.

11. Fear and anxiety that something will happen – an accident.

12. Singing.

13. Laughing.

14. Danger – attack, murder, drowning, death.

15. Injustice, being oppressed, fighting back violently.

16. Feeling alone, helpless, having to fight it out alone there being no one to depend on.

10

THE PROVING OF *POLYSTYRENUM*

A proving of *Polystyrenum* was conducted in February 1995, with ten provers none of whom knew what was being proved. The provers were between the ages of twenty to forty years. They were given one dose each of the substance, in the 30 C potency. Provers G, H and I did not take the proving dose. All the provers were asked to note the symptoms and to meet individually with the master prover once a week. After three weeks, the provers met as a group; during this meeting the symptoms were discussed and the name of the substance finally revealed to them. If any of the provers had any more symptoms after this final meeting, they were asked to get in touch with the master prover; these symptoms have also been incorporated into the proving.

The drug was prepared in the following manner:
– Granules of Polystyrenum were scraped with a nail file. These scraping were triturated upto the 3 C potency using a mortar and pestle. Further potencies upto 30 C were prepared in alcohol, by the Hahnemannian method.

MIND

Emotions

No emotions / Practical

- Practical, able to take immediate, point-blank decisions without getting involved or thinking what the other person would feel; also without any after-thought, like an executive. Felt always that I had done the right thing.

  [A/f/1,*/i]

- Was assertive and non-interfering; quite aloof, detached, objective. Felt others should not get so involved.

  [A/f/1,*/i]

- Cool and collected.

  [A/f/1,*/i]

- No strong emotions, fears.

  [A/f/1,*/i]

- Was angry at a carpenter who had left some work unfinished, and at my mother for being sympathetic and unprofessional.

  [C/m/1,5/i]

- The music that I have been learning and which I could feel in the depths of my soul does not touch me anymore. I think and sing, rather than being involved in the music.

  [C/m/2,*/i]

- No embarrassment in situations that would have earlier been embarrassing.

  [D/m/3,*/i]

- Logical.

  [E/f/*,*/i]

- Absence of the usual irritability when things did not go my way with the feeling that one should let everything happen as and when it wants, and that it wasn't in my control. Was more composed and balanced.

  [J/f/1,*/i]

- Had the feeling,"To hell with savings and all."

  [C/m/*,*/i]

- Lack of my usual hesitation in asking a poor patient for my fees. Charged him with the feeling that people won't value me, if I don't charge more.

  [D/m/2,*/i]

Cleanliness / Order

- In the evenings, a desire to keep things clean and in their proper place, and to have everything in a good appearance.

  [C/m/1,*/i]

- Had the feeling that I should be more organized and methodical in work, make things function in a better way, otherwise everything will be haywire.

  [E/f/before dose]

- Feeling that I have to be more organized more systematic and more careful, especially in money matters.

  [E/f/1,2/i]

- Desire to do a lot of cleaning in the house which I normally postpone.

  [J/f/2,*/i]

Superior / Dominating

- Desire to have a strong and tough

physique. Stick my chest out and clench my fists while walking. Feel very energetic with an inclination to do exercise. Feel like I am the strong and powerful one who will help weaker or disabled people. Felt I could do tough things both physically and mentally and take up jobs which others consider to be difficult.

[C/m/3,*/i]

▪ A feeling, at midnight, that I want to show to the world I am something: "Give me my place, my respect." A craving for success.
[C/m/1,6/i]

▪ Feel like starting a debate with allo-paths, want to show them where they are and where we homoeopaths are. Want that they should agree to our superiority. Hatred towards them.

[C/m/3,*/i]

▪ Wanted to put people in their proper places, to show them where they are.
[I'/f/*,*]

▪ Feel that the person I am conversing with should shut up and listen to me. Curtly dominating.

[C/m/3,*/i]

Enjoyment / Leisure

▪ Recollection of days of enjoyment and fun.
[C/m/2,*/i]

▪ Feeling bored, as if life is dull and monotonous.
[D/m/3,*/i]

▪ Felt I had no sort of pleasure in life.
[J/f/2,*/i]

▪ Tired as if I needed a break. Wanted to go on a holiday and sort out my emotions.
[E/f/3,*/i]

▪ Wanted to read magazines for passing time, rather than study.
[E/f/*,*/i]

▪ Desire to read leisurely material rather than follow my usual, strict routine of studying.
[H'/f/*,*/0]

Used / Usefulness

▪ Felt about a teacher that because he had the controls, he was just using people and students for his own benefit and then discarding them.

[C/m/1,7/i]

▪ Feeling that relationships are mostly selfish and that people try to utilize and take advantage of others; that love and care does not matter but how useful you are or not.

[F/f/*,*/i]

▪ Had the feeling that no one would take me for granted or dominate me, and the person who tried would get a firing from me and I would beat him and pull his hair. I felt that I must be prepared in case anyone tries it.

[D/m/1,4/i]

▪ Sudden thought as to why I was being so considerate, "taking shit" from everyone, taking what they are saying to me without answering.

[I'/f/*,*/0]

Contact / Care

▪ Felt as if all along I have been living with dead people. Now I feel that I am in contact with reality and should get in contact with live people. As if I had been in a dream-world all along.

[J/f/3,*/i]

▪ Needed a lot of cuddling, contact, so that I was sapping out, draining others. As if I had lost someone who was very dear.

[F/f/2,*/i]

▪ Very happy to have come in contact with small children, felt attached to them.

[F/f/2,*/i]

▪ Love contact even with strangers in bus, which I usually do not like and avoid. Badly want close contact with someone of my own. A tremendous desire to travel with

someone very close who would care for me.
[J/f/2,∗/i]

- Expected a lot from others – that they should do things for me and themselves while I sat around, that they should help me, take care of me.

[F/f/∗,∗/i]

- Constant strange feeling of being in a trance, as if my mind and body were separated or as if I wasn't in touch with things around me or with myself. Feeling like there was barrier. Felt as if I was mechanically living my life. Unable to register things I had read.

[F/f/∗,∗/i]

Working / Progressing

- No desire to grow, know more. Not keen regarding career, regarding art or music, of which I was earlier very fond. Instead am affected by daily things, or things happening to people around.

[F/f/2,∗/i]

- Desire to do tough, intellectual work. Tremendous desire to go forward.

[C/m/∗,∗/i]

- Felt I should work harder and somehow increase my income, to meet expenses for which I am solely responsible. Even though there are people who will help me, I don't want to burden them. This is my struggle, my duty (to fulfill what my late father had taken pains to start).

[E/f/1,1/i]

- Feeling that in spite of a lot of hard work, I am not progressing; it is tremendously frustrating. Wanted to stop reading, take a break and rejuvenate myself.

[H'/f/∗,∗/0]

- Strongly started to accept that all changes come through conflicts and peace does not let you grow. If I had to choose between peace and conflict, I would go for conflict.

[F/f/2,∗/i]

Anger / Irritability

- Angry towards the editor of a newspaper which carried a story about the suicide of a homosexual girl. Felt he lacked moral feelings and had put it on the front page only so that the sales of his newspaper would pick up.

[F/f/2,∗/i]

- Anger without repentance.

[J/f/2,∗/i]

- Unusually expressive of my irritability without any remorse.

[I'/f/∗,∗/0]

- Angry, irritable, curt.

[I'/f/∗,∗/0]

- Irritability at children.

[A/f/2,∗/i]

- Irritable, scolding child with desire to strike.

[E/f/3,∗/i]

- Irritable and snappish in the mornings.
[A/f/3,∗/i]

Threats / Fears

- Had the fear that the ferocious dog that was "behind me" might bite me. So thought that I should keep a doberman or a Alsatian dog.

[D/m/1,1/i]

- Had the feeling in the morning that someone would harm me and I should threaten him. But wanted to threaten him only if he was weaker than me. Had the constant fear that some person or group or the police would take me away.

[D/m/1,5/i]

- Feeling of a constant threat of being assaulted, especially by the opposite sex. I felt that it could be anyone, may be even someone from your own family, it may be someone honourable, and it is sudden and from someone you didn't expect. I felt one can't trust anybody, and was treating everyone with suspicion, doubt, fear.

[F/f/∗,∗/i]

- Violent impulses; desire to hit the person ahead of me, while alighting from the train, for being too slow. But a constant fear of the consequences.

[D/m/1,1/i]

- Violence – desire to strike, to clench teeth together. Feeling of being threatened and that I should protect myself by being violent.

[D/m/1,*/i]

Anxiety

- Intermittently get the passing thought that my son should not meet with an accident or should not be kidnapped.

[A/f/2,*/i]

- Anxious and worried about children that something will happen to them.

[A/f/3,*/i]

- Very anxious about child, whether I am looking after her properly or not.

[E/f/before dose]

- Irritable and anxious from the feeling that I was alone and would have to fight out certain situations alone.

[E/f/1,1/i]

- Usual anxiety regarding finances was ameliorated.

[B/m/1,2/i]

Miscellaneous

- Wanted to earn more, have luxuries – a materialistic attitude. Wanted to take up a side-profession simply to earn more.

[F/f/*,*/i]

- A feeling that things I did not expect were happening, that I couldn't trust others, and would lose faith.

[F/f/*,*/i]

- Tried to examine, out of curiosity, how sexual perversions arise in people, right from the embryonic stage, and why homosexuality is commoner amongst males. Felt it is quite normal or natural to have perverted ideas and homosexuality should not be treated as a taboo or looked down upon.

[F/f/2,*/i]

- Interest in human conflicts rather that music or sports. Example: A TV serial that was thought provoking for me involved the son of a widower who had recently found out that his father had been involved with a woman for many years. The boy was very angry, aggressive and began to address his father as Mr. "So and so" rather than "Father". I felt that both reactions were appropriate and that this was a common human problem, whether to behave as society expects you to, or to behave and perform duties to do what you want to. Felt I was able to understand such problems better, and that once I understood them there would be no conflicts left.

[F/f/2,*/i]

- Hurried, others seemed too slow. Impatience with others and myself.

[F/f/*,*/i]

- Time passes too quickly.

[J/f/1,*/i]

- Thinking long before answering.

[C/m/*,*/i]

- Awkward; dropping, toppling, breaking things.

[F/f/*,*/i]

- Seemed more concerned than usual about looks, appearance, especially outlining eyes.

[A/f/*,*/i]

- Desire to change my look: to wear a steel chain (that I used to wear for fashion-shows in the past), and grow a moustache.

[C/m/1,*/i]

- Started to like only white-colored clothes. Marked aversion to red, green and other bright colours.

[J/f/*,*/i]

- Has the sudden thought before falling to sleep, that a glass suddenly broke while in my hand.

[B/m/1,1/i]

- Feel more mature and hopeful.

[C/m/2,∗/i]

- Felt that I should have my independence and freedom.

[D/m/1,4/i]

- Had a lot of determination with the feeling that I will not change against all odds.

[D/m/3,∗/i]

- A song that is constantly in my mind: "Hold me. I will then say to you: 'You are my friend'. Care for me like you are my friend."

[D/m/∗,∗/i]

- Began to listen to pop and rock music (which I have never listened to before).

[J/f/∗,∗/i]

- Felt I was lacking in devotion or communication with God, and that was why my mind was unsteady and wavering. Got much peace from a simple religious ritual.

[E/f/3,∗/i]

- Became critical of a teacher for whom I normally have utmost regard.

[J/f/∗,∗/i]

- Indolence, casual. Aversion physical work.

[H'/m/∗,∗/0]

- Lack of enthusiasm and aims. The "go" has gone out of me.

[H'/m/∗,∗/0]

- Constant desire for company. Talking for hours.

[J/f/1,∗/i]

- A feeling that I am lacking somewhere. I feel that my teachers made a hundred from zero, and that I can't even maintain the hundred. Helpless.

[C/m/∗,∗/i]

- Conflict between what I am doing and what I am supposed to do.

[E/f/1,3/i]

- Violent hateful, revengeful thoughts.

[D/m/1,4/i]

- Conscientiously planning for children's routine.

[A/f/3,∗/i]

- Cheerful in the morning. Depressed in the evening as if from an irreparable loss. Weeping involuntarily at night before going to sleep.

[F/f/2,∗/i]

Intellect

- Dizzy, drugged feeling with inability to concentrate at work and a fear that other cars and persons would bang into me.

[B/m/1,2/i]

- Forgetful, could not recollect what had happened in the morning, whether I had eaten breakfast or not.

[D/m/2,∗/i]

- Dullness of mind, unable to appreciate things, lack precision. Everything seems too hazy. Clarity leads to lack of confidence.

[E/f/2,∗/i]

- Confusion of mind – cannot think clearly. Can't concentrate.

[E/f/3,2/i]

- Sudden clarity of mind about the future, am able to take decisions very quickly. As if suddenly some confusion disappeared, the way is clear, and there is only one path. As if I am able to perceive what is beyond.

[G'/m/1/∗/0]

- A tremendous desire to do intellectual work that will involve skill, knowledge and tension.

[C/m/1,6/i]

DREAMS

Movie actresses

▪ The gate-keeper of a garden that I am entering does not recognize a famous movie actress I am with. I was surprised that such a well-known person can go unnoticed.

[B/m/2,*/i]

▪ Encounter a very famous actress of the yesteryears on the beach. She was a well-known celebrity once upon a time, later she had a psychotic episode and now she is nothing. Remember having been told some-time earlier that she catches hold of people and tells them about how the film industry has taken advantage of her, and troubled her so that she is miserable.

[B/m/2,6/i]

▪ I was amazed to see a famous film actress standing next to me in a public bus. I gave her two rupees with which she bought a ticket with, and returned the change (50 p.) to me.

[C/m/1,2/i]

▪ Enjoying watching a film actress dancing.

[E/f/1,3/i]

▪ Famous movie actress.

[J/f/*,*/i]

No emotions

▪ A monkey falling off a tree. I think casually that it can be eaten up and its tail given to children to play with.

[C/m/1,*/i]

▪ Thin, black wires arranged randomly or in a zig-zag manner, with sparks of white light suddenly appearing in many places, one after the other. No emotions.

[A/f/1,1/i]

▪ Explosion from thumb: mud and rocks flying out. No pain, no emotions.

[A/f/1,1/i]

▪ Indifference to being approached by four men who had the intention to rape me.

[A/f/2,*/i]

▪ Many warplanes were approaching to bomb a building I was standing in, which was very important from the point of view of national security. We were watching it all quite emotionlessly when one of the rockets fell to the ground. We ran over to see it, and found it was unmanned and totally computer-ized. We were discussing fearlessly and with indifference amidst the bombing, that it had been programmed by remote control to blast the building.

[B/m/1,7/i]

▪ I was smoking in the balcony at night when I was alone at home. My parents return-ed suddenly and saw me throw away the cigarette. They were not able to tell me any-thing. I was anxious for a moment, but then surprisingly there was no feeling of guilt. I felt what had happened had happened.

[D/m/2,*/i]

▪ My neighbour is trying to enter while I am bathing. I tell her that she will find me in the condition I was born in. She is embar-rassed and leaves. I did not feel my usual shyness or strong sense of shame.

[D/m/2,*/i]

▪ Awoke with feeling of crude sexuality without any feelings or emotions attached to it.

[I'/f/*,*/0]

▪ About ten or fifteen small, round rats, without the usual fear.

[J/f/3,*/i]

▪ Was on an outing in a religious place, with no religious feeling. I was climbing a wall and had to find some holes in it to put my hands and feet into while climbing. After some distance there were no more holes and

I looked down to see I was not very high.

There was a big hall where boys were making friends with girls; there was no sexual intention, there were just being friends.

Later, our group had split into two; I was with one half on the top of a high building. The others were waiting below as if to get into a boat and were waving 'bye to us, though they were unable to see us. We all began to clap together so that we could let them know where we were.

[B/m/1,4/i]

▪ Was observing, without any religious feeling, a lot of people who had gathered to pray at a temple on the last day of a Hindu festival. There was a lot of activity going on. Later when I passed the place again at midnight, there were people there still, singing religious songs and waiting in a queue for blessings. A patient (I had seen recently) was also in the queue, discussing some problem.

[B/m/1,5/i]

▪ Passing urine with the door of the toilet open. Very embarrassed. I closed the door but later there was no wall. Felt no embarrassment. Told myself to let it be as everyone passes urine.

[J/f/1,2/i]

No privacy

▪ I was with a group of people and a person was showing us his house which was big, majestic, had stained glasses and resembled a European church. Everyone was impressed. Then I took them to my house which was princely, with huge rooms and a lot of furniture. There were new things in it but these seemed out of place. As we came out, there was a big lounge with many chairs in it. I realized that there was a restaurant adjacent to my flat. The two were merged into each other so that there was no clear demarcation between them. I wondered, without any feeling of anxiety, where I would put the door so that people coming to the restaurant wouldn't enter my house.

[B/m/1,6/i]

▪ My house consists of a single room surrounded by two open balconies on either side, so that there is no privacy. Also I realize that there is no ceiling and anyone from the surrounding sky-scrapers can look inside.

[B/m/ after discussing proving]

▪ My conversations were being heard by someone in another room through a microphone. I tear off the microphone with a feeling that I am being spied upon, being watched.

[D/m/2,*/i]

Threat / Danger

▪ A middle-aged man, dressed sophisticatedly in a suit and tie, and for whom I am supposed to be working, is insisting that I stay till late even though I have finished working. Innocently I stay on, but later feel his intentions are sexual and he is trying to touch me without my realizing it. I try to get away.

[F/f/2,*/i]

▪ I am calling out to my brother who is walking ahead of me to come and rescue me as three men come and surround me on the road. He comes to my rescue and the three men go away.

[F/f/2,*/i]

▪ Of being slapped by a patient who had been admitted with a complaint that there was something coming of her legs, and who had been labelled as neurotic. Wanted to take her case although was on guard because of the threat that she might slap me again.

[F/f/2,*/]

▪ Recurrent dream of younger brother embracing me warmly, during some celebration in my honour, and later not leaving me and putting me on a bed. While earlier I had been touched by his gesture, I later felt it was not correct, rather was shameful and embarrassing.

Woke up feeling why am I suffering this sort of dream when my relationship with him is soft, delicate and tender, and he is very dear to me.

If it were to happen in reality, would feel hateful and angry towards him, would not want him around, would lose faith in the relationship, in people – very traumatic. I would always have to be on guard with someone I am always at peace with, safe with, on whom I can rely.

[F/f/2,∗/i]

▪ A very big and long, red truck was being driven by two people. It had to be operated manually rather than with a steering. There seemed to be something mysterious or fishy about it. Then instead of stopping at the signal, it crossed the road-divider and continued going along the opposite side of the road. I feared that if it did not stop it would crush all other vehicles which were smaller and lighter.

[F/f/2,∗/i]

Disgust / Dirty

▪ Something, probably the hand of my younger brother forcefully being thrust into my perineum. Felt pain and disgust.

[F/f/before dose]

▪ Disgust at myself for trying to seduce my close relative.

[H'/m/∗,∗/0]

▪ Lifted up an overturned bowl of food, among many others, to find it contained smashed bananas – the peels and the inner pulp had been separated. Felt "Eeks!" Slimy, dirty feeling!

[A/f/1,∗/i]

▪ A sink full of dirty water with good, whole carrots thrown in. Dirty feeling.

[A/f/1,∗/i]

▪ Crossing a large park which was so dirty in the centre that I thought that the entire city came here to evacuate their bowels. Later, I realized that the periphery was clean and

decided to walk along the clean portion henceforth.

[J/f/∗,∗/i]

▪ Passing stool in a dirty toilet. Dirty embarrassing feeling.

[C/m/1,6/i]

▪ Of falling into a gutter, and a gelatinous, white substance soiling my feet to above the ankles. Feel dirty and disgusted.

[I'/f/∗,∗/0]

Anxious / Fearful

▪ I was offered a cigarette by a family friend whom I met while travelling. He had with him a pack of twenty cigarettes, which he said had cost him sixty rupees. I took a cigarette, folded it lengthwise and was about to light it when I realized, with fear, that this person was known to my family, and I felt I should not smoke.

[D/f/1,i/i]

▪ Trying to escape, with a friend, from someone who was behind me, in the night. We beat him up and wanted to murder him. But because of a fear of being caught, we threw off his body somewhere, having made him unconscious.

[D/f/1,1/i]

▪ I was amongst many people hiding underground in a school hall during a war between India and China. I could see firing all around. Some of us were scared and others were bold; I had the constant fear of being shot but was trying to put up a brave front by keeping myself diverted, doing arcobatics. Then a van and few motorbikes with some chinese militants passed by. All of us were supposed to lie flat on our abdomen with our hands stretched and say, "Hail Zio!" Those who raised their heads were shot.

Inside the school where there were no militants, people were very easy going singing, doing gymnastics and entertaining themselves. Felt that if I was brave I would be mentally sharp and have the presence of mind to act.

[E/f/1,8/i]

■ Fear, on seeing a black monkey outside my kitchen window, that it would enter the house and destroy everything. Ask my brother to shut the window which he does casually so that it re-opens. As I got to shut it again I accidentally touch a water pot that I am not supposed to during my menses. I topples over. I feel bad about my mistake.

[F/f/1,1/i]

■ Recurrent, frightful, vivid dreams of fights and blood, which would awaken me from sleep.

[C/m/1,1/i]

■ I have to undergo surgery for cataract in both my eyes. The tissue from my eyes will then be used for corrective surgery for my baby. The operation of the first eye is successful, after which there is a switch of doctors. The new pair of surgeons is not serious about the operation. They are chatting, entertaining themselves, having a conference in the theatre.

The scene then suddenly changes to a gathering, and one man who is at the back throws a knife, injuring another person.

Then the scene changes back to the operation theatre. I am concerned as to how they will do the operation, and whether my baby will undergo pain from their negligence. I am not so concerned about myself bearing pain. I didn't know what to do.

[E/f/before dose]

■ Astonished that my middle-aged aunt is pregnant, though no one else reacts. Being the only doctor in the family I am supposed to deliver the baby. I am nervous because I lack in experience. But I begin to advise, care for and caution her. I also manage to gather some instruments I would be needing, and which I sterilize. At the last minute the family says that she will deliver in the hospital. I am surprised at the sudden change of decision,

though relieved.

[F/f/before dose]

■ Of being anxious while rejoining an exercise class that I might be expected to be as fit as I had been before.

[E/f/2,3/i]

■ My daughter tells me that my son has been outside in the balcony for a long time and is eating mud. I have to go to get him. I am concerned about my duty towards him.

[A/f/3,*/i]

Colours

■ A bunch of pink flowers.

[C/m/1,6/i]

■ I am visiting a college that is very colourful. I compare it with the college I had attended and feel that it had been colourless, dull and monotonous.

[D/m/2,*/i]

■ Frightful but beautiful dreams, of clusters of many coloured bubbles in an ellipse, swimming in the sky and which are supposed to be chemicals thrown by aliens to destroy the earth.

[J/f/1,*/i]

■ Beautiful dream of walking along a road by the seashore at night with my husband, son, and a friend, and seeing bushes of shaded daisies coloured white and pink. I told my friend that the Earth was very beautiful, and was the Eden of the universe. I said that it is our duty to save it from destruction.

Ahead there was a herd of buffaloes, amongst which five were smaller, and spotted like deer.

[J/f/3,*/i]

Marriage

■ I was in a big hall which was crowded as for a marriage, with a bride, her middle-aged, widowed mother and the groom who was presumably my older brother. As I walked through the ceremonies with them, I had the feeling that I was the one being married to the girl. But to my surprise I realized at the end of it all that I had been married to the widow and my brother to the girl. I felt that in some way my brother was smart, had done things well.

[B/m/1,6/i]

- Marriage ceremony.

[E/f/1,2/i]

- Recurrent dreams of weddings.

[J/f/3,*/i]

- Two of my old schoolmates with whom I wasn't very well acquainted came to my house and arrogantly asked me to leave the place and to send my mother. I was surprised; they don't usually speak to me and now they are being so arrogant. They were talking amongst themselves as if one of them intended to propose marriage to me; he was saying that he was an engineer from U.S.A.

[F/f/1,1/i]

Teachers

- I was being shouted at by my teacher for being unable to answer the question he had asked me. He was telling me that I didn't know a thing and was commenting on the way I talk. I felt hurt at what he said and was totally disappointed because I didn't know anything. I felt dull amongst a class of bright students, as if I was nothing. I began to borrow books from my friends to read with the feeling that I have to grow, and cannot stagnate.

[E/f/3,*/i]

- My professor left the class very upset because I had yawned when he said he was going to talk about the Ammonium group. I went after him to tell him it was not intended, that it was merely an accident and that he should come back and teach. But I was unable to catch up with him. I felt bad that the entire class would suffer because of my mistake.

[F/f/before dose]

- Chatting with my professor at a function in a hilly area. It was night-time and he was surrounded by a lot of people. Then I had to stay with a friend in a jungle-like area. I come to know his remedy is *Staphysagria*.

[D/m/1,4/i]

- A very attractive, small snake with blue and white markings was kept in a glass container in a hall. Many people had gathered there for a lecture. I was having a friendly conversation with a teacher for whom I usually feel a respectful fear. Later, I went for a drive with him in an open car, on his suggestion. I was advising him to buy a house in a posh area.

[C/m/1,3/i]

- A lecturer was telling us about a new theory of case analysis where each case had to be divided into six steps. Of these, the first step involved knowing the onset, depth and chronicity of the complaint and the second step involved knowing the miasm. From amongst all the people present there only I did not know about the theory, and was asking her questions for clarification in reply to which she was giving a brief explanation.

[D/m/1,2/i]

Friends

- Was in a car riding with two friends – one was talking to me while the other was driving the car. Felt about the driver, that he was being neglected, that he has kept like a chauffeur, and that we were wasting his time. I felt thet he may be busy and that we should let him go.

[F/f/1,2/i]

- My friends had dropped in early in the morning on my birthday, with bouquets. I thought they were very caring to have come so early, but after they left I began to wonder whether they just treated it as a formality and wanted to finish it off early so that it doesn't disturb their normal routine.

[F/f/2,*/i]

- I am beating up a friend and feeling very happy.

[D/m/3,*/i]

- Pleasant dreams of being amongst a group of friends.

[J/f/*,*/i]

- Meeting an old friend.

[D/m/1,*/i]

- My friend had fallen off the terrace of a building. I was unconscious from typhoid and when I woke up after three days, I enquired about him. I was saddened when I was told that he had died.

About the friend: He used to be a reporter, wants more university degrees, to study more. Although people think he is great, he is just like any other person; is egoless. He appeared on television very often. Has tremendous will power – lost forty kilos in one year through very strict diet, very long walks. Timid. He talks to everyone with a lot of respect. Junior most, but most respected officer. In spite of having a good rank, and being given beautiful house (like a bungalow in Switzerland), he goes on picnics with us. He shaves only once or twice a year, and when he does, he also shaves his head. He is indifferent to his personal appearance. At other times he keeps his hair and beard long. He likes music, old classical music which normal people will not understand.

He is twenty-seven years old, yet unmarried (unusual for an Indian of his status). Has good relations with ministers of government. Knows about astrology. Had bought only two clothes in the entire five and a half years of college, although he is very rich. He will wear a shirt instead of a coat in a photo session, yet his photograph is the best. There is logic behind everything he says: for example, he believes that the caste system followed in rural India has a function in society, as has been explained in ancient Indian texts (Vedas).

[D/m/3,*/i]

Miscellaneous

- A woman with a peculiar, horrible face that had one eye smaller than the other, and one side bandaged while the other part was good.

[A/f/1,*/i]

- Of telling a strange woman that where there is a will there is a way.

[D/m/2,*/i]

- My mother's friends had given me a lot of valuable gifts on the occasion of my starting my own clinic. They were mostly perfumes, things made of glass, that were expensive and delicate, that one wouldn't use in everyday life but would preserve. I decide to keep them away and put them into a toilet which is apart from the house. Then I feel that someone might rob or snatch them away and decide to put them back into the house. I call two cousins to help me by taking things back to the house while I wait at the toilet. But once in the house, they get busy with their own work and I am still waiting for them. After waiting long I go back to the house and am terribly angry at them for fooling me and keeping me waiting while they are busy in their own work.

[C/m/1,6/i]

- My old grandmother (dead) has been made to sit in a separate room and watch the celebrations for my brothers wedding through the window, because there is too much of a crowd outside. I feel very bad that she has to be kept separate and that she cannot enjoy the celebrations. She used to do anything and everything for everybody but was asked by her children to get out. She was very fastidious, loved money and gold.

Later my mother who was busy gave me a small baby to hold.

[J/f/3,*/i]

- My hair has all turned grey and I feel that there are no chances of my getting married now. Then I tell myself that it didn't matter since I had accepted the idea long ago, and so I shouldn't bother. Instead I feel I should just relax and go back to bed.

I observe my hair again and then realize that it is black from the outside. When I pick out a lock I see that it is totally white from the inside and so resembles the wing of a bird.

[I'/f/after discussing proving]

■ An officer who had been a college friend has greyed, and was being taken in a wheelchair on the college campus. I thought he may have met with an accident. But as he approached the hospital, he got out of the wheelchair.

[D/m/1,3/i]

■ My children were giving a swimming test in a river that ran through a place of pilgrimage. They were shouting to me to watch them swim across. I wondered how the woman taking their test was going to stay the duration of the test (three days and three nights) in the water.

[B/m/1,5/i]

■ Performing a religious ritual with parents.

[J/f/2,*/i]

■ Was observing a lot of Muslim people going up the hall to a mosque, and praying, performing religious rituals.

[B/m/1,5/i]

■ Explaining where the entrance of my clinic (which was being renovated) will be.

[B/m/1,3/i]

■ I am watching a train move away from the platform when there is a sudden shriek from the ladies compartment. Everyone's attention is diverted there and the train stops. The driver and everyone around want to know if anyone is in distress and needs help. Then they realize that there is nothing the matter and the train moves away.

[D/m/2,*/i]

■ Met with an accident with a cyclist while driving slowly.

[A/f/2,*/i]

■ Of going downhill while driving with my son, and meeting with an accident.

[A/f/2,*/i]

■ Was at the railway station when it was announced that some changes had been made in the stations and the number of railways tracks for the convenience of commuters. The train that was to arrive at my platform stopped on another platform, and a second train also arrived, again on another platform. I was in a hurry to board the train but could not cross tracks as the bridge was too far away.

Then I began to converse with a man polishing shoes who sympathized with me.

[D/m/1,4/i]

■ My father-in-law was counselling me not to sell off some gold jewellery as I had been planning in order to clear a loan. Then some relatives showed up who volunteered to lend me money to clear the loan.

[B/m/1,6/i]

■ My son was going on eating a lot of biscuits. I felt he should be trained.

[B/m/1,5/i]

■ Was feeling, while standing in a usually crowded subway, that a lot of discipline was required here, otherwise there would be chaos.

[B/m/1,5/i]

■ Embarrassing dream of changing in a friends house while the window was open so that other people could look inside.

[J/f/1,*/i]

■ The manager of a supermarket is examining the contents of my shirt pocket, while I am unloading the things I intend to buy at the counter. He finds an old pencil sharpener in my pocket, and accuses me of having picked it up from the supermarket and not wanting to pay for it. I am very offended, and ashamed that he is saying this in front of others. I am supposed to be well-known and trusted in the place. I did not argue because

I felt, it was no point to do so.

[G'/m/1,*/0]

- Of being criticized or accused wrongly of doing something.

[G'/m/1,*/0]

- The brother of a "gangster-type of person" is inquiring about my practice.

[D/f/1,*/i]

- Vivid dream of fighting with and angrily abusing a carpenter who hadn't finished a task I had given him; shouting at him in a very loud voice.

[C/m/3,*/i]

- Horses on a merry-go-round.

[A/f/2,6/i]

- Embraced affectionately by nephew when I returned home from a foreign country. I felt affectionate towards him and played with him.

[C/m/1,2/i]

- My mother was receiving a lot of guests at a big function.

[F/f/1,1/i]

- Cooking for children.

[A/f/3,*/i]

- My son had scored poorly, and I had to take the favour from someone I had been fighting with to get him into college. A friend tells me I shouldn't have trusted this person and that he would get my son into any other college.

[J/f/2,*/i]

- Walking along a beach.

[B/m/1,4/i]

- Showing my house to two German visitors.

[C/m/1,7/i]

- My sister is engaged, and is complaining that her in-laws are strict and that she is not allowed to eat in restaurants.

[D/m/2,*/i]

- I had been informed that a group discussion was to be held at my house and was searching frantically for something appropriate to wear. I found some clothes but they were not to my satisfaction, so I changed. I was hurried because the group might arrive anytime. Later, I was informed that no one would come and felt that after going through all the hurry, there was nothing in the end.

[F/f/3,*/i]

- Woke up with a jerk as if I was falling off the last step of a staircase.

[J/f/2,4/i]

- I had attended a religious function at the end of which we were given batata-wadas [1]. My husband was given a bigger one. I felt they have given me a smaller one because I would put on weight.

[J/f/3,*/i]

- Dancing for hours together.

[J/f/*,*/i]

- I am standing in front of the Parliament House. I am thinking to myself that a civil servant who is helping my room-mate appear for the civil services exam can also help me to appear.

(I want to be like this civil servant. About him: Always top ranking. People think he is great. Can give any exam without previous preparation.)

[D/m/*,*/i]

- Fruits.

[J/f/1,*/i]

- Trees with many ripe guavas which had been cut off and put into a truck.

[J/f/1,*/i]

---

[1]   Fried Indian snack, made from potatoes.

STRANGE PHENOMENA OR CO-INCIDENCES DURING THE PROVING

• Seem to be coming in contact with a lot of chain smokers and alcoholics, and also a lot of honest persons who constantly talk about crimes and courts.

[J/f/2,*/i]

• Was full of admiration towards a prominent public figure towards whom I had no such feeling earlier. Compared him to a previous powerful prime minister and thought that the country needed someone as worthy as him, with a very strong will and very good performance.

[D/m/*,*/i]

PHYSICAL SYMPTOMS

Generalities

• Malaise.

[B/m/1,*/i]

• Tired in the mornings. No desire to get out of bed.

[C/m/1,6/i]

• Tiredness, with bodyache.

[D/m/*,*/i]

• Extreme prostration, wanted to lie down and do nothing.

[E/f/before dose]

• Bodyache during menses.

[E/f/*,*/i]

• Chilly, aversion to draft of air.

[E/f/*,*/i]

• Pain in dependent parts as if inflamed.

[E/f/*,*/i]

• Periodicity of complaints; aggravated weekly and on every fourth day.

[F/f/*,*/i]

• Evening aggravation.

[F/f/*,*/i]

• Desires apples.

[J/f/2,*/i]

• Decreased desire for sweets and chocolates, grapes, chilled drinks, of which I am usually fond.

[J/f/2,*/i]

• Desires bhelpuri, pani puri.

[E/f/*,*/i]

Physical particulars

Vertigo

• Dizziness – unable to concentrate.

[B/m/1,2/i]

Head

• Heaviness.

[A/f/1,*/i]

• Severe, throbbing pain in left temporal and supra-orbital regions in the morning. Ameliorated in the afternoon. Unable to read or engage in any activity from the pain.

[A/f/2,*/i]

• Dull pain and heaviness in supra-orbital and temporal regions. A caught-up feeling around the eyes and in the face in the evenings.

[B/m/1,*/i]

- Terrible pain, worse in the evening and night, and better in the morning.

[C/m/1,*/i]

- Heaviness in frontal sinuses. Pain between 11 a.m. and 2.30 p.m., left- sided, with a desire to lie down.

[E/f/2,*/i]

- Throbbing headache in temples, worse from noise.

[E/f/3,*/i]

Eyes

- Dull pain in the eyeballs in the morning, as if strained.

[B/m/1,*/i]

- Burning in the eyes.

[D/m/1,*/i]

- Agglutination of lids, and sticky discharge.

[D/m/1,4/i]

- Foreign body sensation in the right eye.

[E/f/2,*/i]

Ears

- Sounds in ears; sudden, buzzing.

[B/m/1,4/i]

- Heat in ears; worse talking, exertion.

[C/m/1,*/i]

Nose / Smell

- Purulent discharge from right nostril, greenish yellow.

[B/m/1,*/i].

- Sneezing in the morning.

[B/m/1,*/i]

- Colds with yellow discharge.

[D/m/*,*/i]

Face

- Left-sided maxillary sinusitis restarted.

[A/f/*,*/i].

- Sinusitis; dull, caught-up feeling around the eyes, zygomatic process and temples, in the evening.

[C/m/*,*/i].

Mouth

- Itching in the upper palate.

[E/f/2,*/i].

Throat

- Choking, constrictive sensation in trachea restarted.

[B/m/1,*/i]

- Sensation as of a bunch of hair in the throat, which I have to clear.

[C/f/1,1/i]

- Sensitive spot in throat. Raw, sore pain in the morning, aggravated from swallowing.

[D/m/1,*/i]

- Constant soreness in throat, ameliorated from warmth of hand.

[D/m/2,*/i]

- Right-sided cervical node enlarged, painless.

[D/m/2,*/i].

- Irritation in the throat.

[D/m/*,*/i]

- Must clear the throat often.

[E/f/2,*/i]

- Rattling mucus in throat, with cough.

[E/f/2,*/i]

Stomach

- Loud belching.

[D/m/1,1/i]

- Nausea, water brash, worse after eating.

[D/m/1,2/i]

- Dull, aching, epigastric pain.

[D/m/1,1/i]

- Nausea throughout the day.

[E/f/before dose]

- Tremendous thirst (for Pepsi).

[E/f/*,*/i]

- Sudden hunger.

[E/f/*,*/i]

- Nausea from sight of food, worse before meals.

[F/f/*,*/i]

- Gripping pain in abdomen.

[F/f/*,*/i]

- Appetite decreased.

[J/f/1,*/i]

- Appetite: very hungry, but eat a few mouthfuls.

[J/f/2,*/i]

- Loss of appetite, and nausea.

[F/f/2,*/i]

Rectum

- Constipation.

[E/f/1,*/i]

Urinary organs

- Burning in urethra.

[D/m/1,1/i]

Female

- Premenstrual spotting for one or two days before menses, then no flow for two days, followed by regular menses.

[A/f/1,*/i]

- Menses very heavy, accompanied by indolence.

[J/f/2,*/i]

Respiratory

- Sudden attack of my usual asthma, with aching in the back. Was very chilly before and after midnight, during the attack. [The prover had a history of breathlessness and last suffered from an asthamatic attack six months prior to the proving].

[D/m/2,*/i]

- Breathlessness, feel better until 4.00 p.m., then gradually begins. Ameliorated in the knee-elbow position, lying on back.

[H'/m/*,*/0]

Back

- Dull aching pain in sacral region, which later extended to the legs.

[C/m/1,*/i]

- Backache, with unusual stiffness in the middle and lower back. Aggravated on waking. Ameliorated in the daytime.

[E/f/*,*/i]

- Aching in the back, with breathlessness.

[H'/m/*,*/0]

- Severe backpain with menses.

[E/f/2,*/i]

- Backpain, worse on the side laid on.

[J/f/2,*/i]

Chest

- Heaviness in the chest at night.

[C/m/*,*/i]

- Retrosternal burning.

[D/m/1,1/i]

- Heaviness in the chest.

[E/f/2,*/i]

Expectoration

- Yellow, stringy.

[D/m/2,*/i]

Cough

- Cough, aggravated 7.00 p.m. - 8.00 p.m., of sudden onset.

[D/m/2,*/i]

- Cough, worse in the morning, after brushing teeth.

[E/f/3,*/i]

Extremities

- Constant pain in the legs, especially in the morning, behind the knees.

[D/m/*,*/i].

- Aching pain in the hollow of the knees and in the medial aspect of the knee joint, constant and nagging.

[D/m/*,*/i]

• Palms and feet icy cold, as if washed in water.

[D/m/*,*/i]

• Aching pain in the legs, especially the left leg, behind knees.

[E/f/1,*/i]

• Constant nagging in the ankles.

[E/f/1,*/i]

• Hands and feet icy cold in the evening.

[E/f/*,*/i]

• Oedema feet, right more than left.

[E/f/*,*/i]

• Cramps in the right foot, lateral aspect.

[E/f/*,*/i]

• Neuralgic pain, left heel to femoral canal.

[E/f/*,*/i]

Sleep

• Unable to sleep from heaviness in the chest and activity of mind.

[C/m/1,6/i]

Skin

• Old, itching eruptions on skin reappeared.

[C/m/1,*/i]

• Suppuration of abrasion.

[D/m/1,5/i]

RUBRICS

Mind

Single symptoms
— Ambition, loss of, trifles, affected, by.
— Anger, sympathy and unprofessiona-
lism, from.
— Casual.
— Confusion, emotions, about.
— Contact, desire for.
— Contact, desire for, reality and real
people, with.
— Decisions, easy.
— Decisions, practical.
— Delusion, barrier, not in touch with
things around her, nor with herself.
— Delusion, dominated, he is.
— Delusion, granted, being taken for.
— Delusion, haywire, things going.
— Delusion, selfish, others are.
— Delusion, used and discarded, being.
— Delusion, valued, he is not.
— Dreams, aliens destroying the earth.
— Dreams, animals, buffaloes, spotted.
— Dreams, animals, monkey, black.
— Dreams, animals, monkey, utilized as
food and plaything.
— Dreams, animals, snakes, blue and
white.
— Dreams, body, bodyparts, hair greying.
— Dreams, bombs falling.
— Dreams, chaos.
— Dreams, clusters of colourful bubbles
in the sky.
— Dreams, college, colourful.
— Dreams, convenience, being unable to
utilize.
— Dreams, daisies.

— Dreams, doctors, neglectful.
— **Dreams, emotions, without**.
— Dreams, explosions, thumb, of.
— Dreams, faces, horrible.
— Dreams, friends, beating up his friend,
happy to be.
— Dreams, friends, treating her birthday
as a formality.
— Dreams, friends, chauffeur, friend was
being used as.
— Dreams, grandmother, old, isolated.
— Dreams, helping persons in distress.
— Dreams, isolated, of being.
— Dreams, incest.
— Dreams, houses, majestic.
— Dreams, house, door, without.
— Dreams, house, privacy, without.
— *Dreams, movie actresses*.
— Dreams, movie actresses, advantage
being taken of.
— Dreams, movie actress, money, lend-
ing to.
— Dreams, movie actress, recognize,
failing to.
— Dreams, murder, disposing of corpse.
— Dreams, rape, threat of, indifferent to.
— Dreams, rocket, unmanned, computer-
ized.
— Dreams, shocking events, emotions,
without.
— Dreams, spied upon, watched, being.
— Dreams, truck, big, red, crushing
smaller, lighter vehicles.
— Dreams, valuable, delicate objects,
preserving, of.

— Dreams, weddings, tricked into marrying a widow.
— Dreams, wires, sparking, randomly arranged.
— Emotions, absent, sexual desire, with.
— Fear.
— Intellectual work, desire for.
— *Involvement, reduced.*
— Involvement, reduced, practical, logical behaviour.
— Listened to, desires to be.
— Looks, concerned about his.
— Materialistic.
— Monotonous, feeling.
— Organized and methodical, desires to be.
— Remorse, want of.
— Sadness, melancholy, loss, irreparable, as from.
— Sexual perversions.
— Success, craves, demands his place and respect.
— Surprises, shocks, unaffected by.
— Suspicious, men, about.
— Threatened, feels.
— Tough, desire to be.

Common symptoms
— Abrupt.
— Ambition, loss of.
— Ambition increased.
— Amusement, desire for.
— Anger, irascibility.
— Answers, reflects long.
— Answers, snappishly.
— Anxiety, children, about his.
— Automatic gestures.
— Awkward, drops things.
— Censorious, critical.

— Cheerfulness, morning.
— Colours, green, aversion to.
— Colours, red, aversion to
— Colours, white, desire for.
— Company, desire for.
— Concentration, difficult.
— Confidence, want of self.
— Contemptous.
— Delusion, injury, about to receive,
— Delusion, separated, mind and body, are.
— Delusion, superiority, of.
— Determination.
— Dictatorial, domineering.
— Dreams, accidents.
— Dreams, accusations, wrongfully accused of a crime.
— Dreams, affectionate.
— Dreams, animals.
— Dreams, animals, rats.
— Dreams, anxious.
— Dreams, beautiful.
— Dreams, closet, being on.
— Dreams, anxious.
— Dreams, blood.
— Dreams, dancing.
— Dreams, danger.
— Dreams, dirty.
— *Dreams, disgusting.*
— *Dreams, embarrassment.*
— Dreams, excrements.
— Dreams, excrements, wading in excrements.
— Dreams, falling.
— Dreams, fighting.
— Dreams, fleeing.
— Dreams, friends, old.
— Dreams, fruits.

— Dreams, houses, big.
— Dreams, mistakes, of making.
— Dreams, money, gold, of.
— Dreams, people, crowds of.
— Dreams, pursued, being.
— Dreams, shameful.
— Dreams, stools.
— Dreams, vivid.
— Dreams, wars.
— Dreams, weddings.
— Dullness, sluggishness.
— Fear, dogs, of.
— Forsaken feeling, sensation of isolation.
— Hatred.
— Helplessness, feeling of.
— Hurry, haste.
— Impatience, slowly, everything goes too.
— Impatience, working, while.
— Indifference.
— Indifference, everything, to
— Indifference, external things, to.
— Indifference, music, which he loves, to.

— Indolence, aversion to work.
— Irritability, morning.
— Irritability, children towards.
— Loquacity.
— Malicious.
— Memory, weakness of.
— Moral, feeling, want of.
— Pertinacity.
— Plans, makes many.
— Religious affections
— Rudeness.
— Sadness, melancholy, evening,
— Striking.
— Succeeds never.
— Suspicious, mistrustful.
— Thoughts, clearness of.
— Time, quickly, appears shorter, passes, too.
— Violent, vehement.
— Weeping, tearful mood, night.
— Weeping, involuntary.
— Wills, two will, sensation as if he has.
— Work, mental, aversion to.
— Work, mental, desires.

PHYSICAL SYMPTOMS

Generalities
– Evening.
– Air, draft aggravates.
– Cold, aggravates.
– Food and drink, apples, desires.
– Menses, during, aggravates.
– Pain.
– Pain, parts, lain on, in.
– Periodicity, day, fourth.

– Periodicity, week, every.
– Weakness
– Weakness, morning, bed, in.
– Weariness.

Vertigo
– Vertigo.

Head
– Constriction.
– Constriction, evening.

- Constriction, forehead, eyes, over.
- Heaviness.
- Heaviness, forehead, eyes, above (single).
- Heaviness, temples.
- Pain.
- Pain, morning, 11.00 a.m., 2.30 p.m., until (single).
- Pain, morning ameliorates.
- Pain, evening.
- Pain, night.
- Pain, lie down, must.
- Pain, sides, left.
- Pain, dull, left.
- Pain, dull pain, forehead, eyes, over.
- Pain, dull pain, temples.
- Pulsating.
- Pulsating, morning.
- Pulsating, afternoon ameliorates (single).
- Pulsating, reading, while sitting.
- Pulsating, forehead, eyes, over.
- Pulsating, temples.
- Pulsating, temples, left.
- Pulsating, temples, noise, from (single).

Eyes
- Agglutinated.
- Discharges, viscid.
- Pain, aching, morning.
- Pain, burning.

Ears
- Heat in.
- Heat, exertion aggravates (single).
- Heat, talking aggravates (single).
- Noises, buzzing.
- Discharge, one side, right.
- Discharge, greenish.
- Discharge, purulent.

- Discharge, yellow.
- Sneezing, morning.

Face
- Pain, evenings.
- Pain, cheeks.
- Pain, zygoma.

Mouth
- Itching, palate.

Throat
- Choking.
- Hair, sensation, of a.
- Irritation.
- Lump, sensation, of a.
- Pain, rawness, morning.
- Pain, rawness, swallowing, when.
- Pain, sore.
- Pain, sore, morning.
- Pain, sore, spot, in a.
- Pain, sore, warmth, external, ameliorates (single).
- Swallowing difficult.

External throat
- Swelling, cervical glands.

Stomach
- Appetite diminished.
- Appetite, easy satiety.
- Appetite, increased
- Appetite, ravenous, easy satiety.
- Eructations, loud
- Eructations, water brash.
- Nausea.
- Nausea, daytime.
- Nausea, eating, before.
- Nausea, eating, after.
- Nausea, food, looking at.
- Pain.

Abdomen
- Pain, cramping.

Rectum
- Constipation.

Urethra
- Pain, burning.

Female
- Menses, copious.

Respiratory
- Difficult.
- Difficult, afternoon, 4.00 p.m., after (single).
- Difficult, accompanied by back pain.
- Difficult, lying back ameliorates.
- Difficult, lying, knees and elbows, ameliorates, on.

Cough
- Cough, morning.
- Cough, evening, 7.00 p.m.
- Cough, evening, 8.00 p.m.
- Cough, rinsing mouth aggravates.
- Cough, sudden.

Expectoration
- Stringy.
- Yellow.

Chest
- Oppression.
- Oppression, nights.
- Pain, burning, sternum, behind.

Back
- Pain.
- Pain, morning, waking, on.
- Pain, lying, while, side, on.
- Pain, menses, during.
- Pain, pressure.
- Pain, aching.

- Pain, aching, sacrum, extending into lower extremities.

Extremities
- Coldness, hands.
- Coldness, hands, evening.
- Coldness, hands, icy.
- Coldness, foot.
- Coldness, foot, evening.
- Coldness, foot, icy cold.
- Cramps, foot, right.
- Cramps, foot, outside of.
- Pain, neuralgic.
- Pain, knee, hollow of.
- Pain, legs, morning.
- Pain, ankle.
- Pain, heel, extending into leg (single).
- Pain, aching.
- Pain, aching, knee, hollow of.
- Pain, aching, leg.
- Pain, aching, leg, left.
- Swelling, foot.
- Swelling, foot, right.

Sleep
- Sleeplessness, oppression in chest, from (single).
- Sleeplessness, thoughts, activity of thoughts, from.

Skin
- Itching.
- Eruptions, suppurating.

THEMES

1. No feeling, no involvement. Practical. No positive or negative feelings. No feeling of participation.

2. Everything should be in its place.

3. Something expensive and delicate which has to be preserved and not used in everyday life.

4. Dirty, disgusting feeling.

5. I am not going to be taken for granted. Hatred towards people who take me for granted.

6. Give me my place, my respect. Well-known actress coming down to an ordinary position.

7. Need for too much contact with friends.

8. Sudden change and surprise, things are happening and suddenly something else happens.

9. No embarrassment in situations of guilt and embarrassment.
   Too much embarrassment.
   No feeling from threat of rape.

10. I can't face the situation if I have fear, but only if I am brave.

11. Emotionless, practical way. Should have the presence of mind, be sharp.

12. Person who is popular with people. Wins awards without preparation. Many degrees in various disciplines. Humble though others think he is great. Tremendous will: lost weight by eating same food for one year. Indifference to appearance. Egoless.

13. Grandmother being kept separate from other because she is of no use. One just uses others for their own benefit. Well-known actress says, she was used by the film industry.

14. When one is in trouble, everyone cares for that person.

15. Money, materialistic.

16. Indolence, lack of ambition.
    Ambition. Desire for tough intellectual work.

11

THE PROVING OF *STRONTIUM CARBONICUM*

The proving of *Strontium carbonicum* was conducted in December 1994, with ten provers. They were roughly between the ages of twenty and thirty years. At the first meeting each prover received one proving dose of the substance in the 30 C potency, with instructions to observe and note down all mental and physical symptoms, dreams, and other peculiar and strange phenomena that he or she experienced. All the provers took the dose. They reported to me individually once a week for the next four weeks. At the end of four weeks, the provers met with me as a group, collectively discussed their symptoms, and the proving was concluded when I revealed the name of the remedy to them. If any of them continued to have symptoms, they were asked to get in touch with me and such symptoms have also been added into this proving.

The drug was obtained from the Pharmacy "Roy and Company", Bombay.

MIND

Emotions

Behind him

- While lying on my side at night had the fear as if some hand would come from behind and do harm to me. So I tried to lie on my back. Fear increased so much that I asked my mother if I could sleep next to her. It took very long to fall asleep when I was alone. Fear of darkness also.

[H/f/1,1/i]

- Constant fear as if someone is following me, as if the person behind me will harm me, or say something bad. Fear of going into lonely place by myself; feel as if some one will come and hurt me. Have become suspicious of people around me when in a public place.

[H/f/3,*/i]

- Caught hold of a person by his shirt and started to scold him when he repeatedly pushed me from behind.

[C/f/1,4/i]

- Anxiety about the future has lessened since assurances from one of my professors. I feel sincere and responsible. Feel as if I have some support behind me, someone to give me guidelines about the future, about the profession. I feel I need it because there is no doctor in my family. I need someone to help me out because I am new to the profession, and will face difficulties. This was the first time I have had a discussion with my professor about setting up practice. I feel he has sound knowledge, respect him for it, and feel

he is a good person to guide me.

[G/m/*,*/i]

- Feel my friends will do something behind me. I trust them but have no guarantee that they will not break the faith.

[A/m/1,6/i]

Friends / Company

- I felt that I could understand my friends' problems better and I am always in contact with a friend who is in trouble or who has problem. My friend was very nervous, and so I was nervous and restless because I thought I have the same problem and I can understand his feelings better than other people. Felt I was experiencing the same things as him.

[A/m/1,5/i]

- Feel that my friends are faithful and that I must not break this faith that I want.

[A/m/1,6/i]

- I felt my friend didn't want to talk to me; I felt unwanted by her. I had the feeling that she was trying to put me down in some way. I began to feel that one should never have many friends; they are not faithful and they always try to cheat you. I felt that I was better off with one best friend who was faithful and I shouldn't bother to even talk to the others. Was depressed and didn't talk to anyone.

[F/f/1,2/i]

- Desire for company, but do not like

crowds. So I sat with just one friend, but away from the rest of my group.

[D/f/1,1/i]

- Don't care for relationships anymore (earlier wanted to maintain relationships).

[D/f/2,*,i]

- Very angry when I felt that my friends were being selfish. Shouted at them. Was not satisfied with their apologies.

[F/f/1,3/i]

- Felt that my friends were suspicious of me, that they would cheat me. Later, felt that I will not bother about it.

[A/m/1,7/i]

- Usual desire for company was reduced. It doesn't matter if family or friends leave me (normally, sensitive to being left alone).

[D/f/1,3/i]

- Happy, talkative with friends.

[I/m/1,2/i]

- Strong desire for company. Feel very lonely.

[D/f/2,*/i]

- Was very nervous when I could not keep a promise I had made to my friends. Fear what they would say.

[I/m/2,2/i]

- "Shy" about what my friends would have said about me when I left a game I wasn't playing very well at.

[I/m/1,3/i]

- Had to suppress my anger when a friend insulted me because I felt I needed to maintain the friendship.

[I/m/*,*/i]

- Didn't feel like talking to anyone. Was not my usual talkative and jovial self. Wanted to stay alone. Was feeling depressed.

[F/f/1,1/i]

- Feel I don't need to talk to a close friend I quarrelled with (earlier friends meant everything for me.)

[C/f/2,*/i]

- Like to remain alone. Don't like to talk with anyone.

[I/m/1,1/i]

- Developed a hatred for some friends; can't bear the look of them.

[F/f/2,*/i]

- Developed a tendency to help my friends, because I feel they will also help me.

[I/m/1,2/i]

Contradiction / Opposition

- The slightest thing against my wish causes me to become very nervous.

[B/m/1,7/i]

- Wanted to do things in my own way. Could not bear any contradiction.

[C/f/1,7/i]

- Very irritable from trifles, very angry and quarrelsome with family members. Anger from opposition or when someone disagrees. Become quiet from anger, unable to speak a right word. Feel I am in the right. Want to beat them.

[D/f/1,2/i]

- Was able to oppose people (am normally yielding).

[H/f/2,*/i]

- Didn't want to oppose a man who was saying bad things about me. Remained quiet and only heard what he had to say.

[I/m/1,1/i]

Irritability / Anger

- Was angry, quarrelsome and refused to eat because the dinner wasn't to my liking.

[F/f/1,1/i]

- Easily irritable.

[D/f/1,3/i]

- Suppressed my anger.

[B/m/1,7/i]

- Irritable from slightest noise. Very sensitive to noise. Couldn't bear anyone talking.

[C/f/1,3/i]

- Angry from noise.

[D/f/1,1/i]

- Changeable moods. Sometime was irritable at "non-specific" things, otherwise in a good mood.

[B/m/1,3/i]

- Usual irritability was ameliorated.

[I/m/1,2/i]

Enjoyment / Amusement

- Felt unhappy, wanted to watch a movie. Very happy to watch it, but felt I had wasted time afterwards.

[A/m/1,4/i]

- Wanted to enjoy myself watching movies, going to different places, spending money on T-shirts and cards. Spent much more than I usually do. Was bunking lectures. Wanted to see different places, to travel.

[C//2,1/i]

- Averse to joining friends for a film, an activity I usually enjoy.

[I/m/1,3/i]

- Anxiety regarding future – how will I be able to study. Forgot the anxiety an hour later, and wanted to enjoy myself.

[A/m/1,6/i]

Restlessness

- Restlessness, physical.

[B/m/2,2/i]

- Restlessness, mental; worse after 4.00 p.m.

[B/m/2,3/i]

- Apologized to a friend who shouted at me without reason. Later felt mentally restless, but wanted to sit down. Angry that I had suppressed my anger, that I did not show my anger to other people, and didn't want the quarrel to go further. Felt better after 4.30 p.m., not restless anymore.

[B/m/1,1/i]

- Feeling restless since last week. Cannot do one thing completely.

[A/m/1,5/i]

- Hurried, impulsive.

[H/f/1,*/i]

Miscellaneous

- Depression, do not like anything, from thinking about the future.

[D/f/1,3/i]

- Hearing strange sounds at night.

[G/m/1,4/i]

- Fear of robbers; locked doors and windows well.

[G/m/1,1/i]

- Want to curse and abuse, though do not actually do it.

[H/f/1,4/i]

- Rudeness in speech. Sensitivity reduced.

[D/f/1,2/i]

- Wanted to hear music all the while.

[F/f/2,2/i]

- Liked music.

[H/f/1,3/i]

- Liked to write.

[H/f/1,3/i]

- Conflict, felt the need for a girlfriend, but a sense of responsibility stopped me. Felt that it wasn't the time now.

[G/m/1,2/i]

- Selfish. Don't care for anyone.

[D/f/1,3/i]

- Have become self-centred.

[G/m/*,*/i]

- Selfish behaviour and attitude.

[H/f/1,5/i]

- Absence of usual anticipatory anxiety about keeping time.

[H//1,5/i]

- Usual anxiety before any task or performance was much less. Was able to perform my work coolly.

[C/f/2,2/i]

- Fear, before taking the dose, as if something would happen.

[H/f/before dose]

- Revengeful, tit-for-tat attitude.
  [H/f/3,∗/i]

- Revengeful. People have to pay for what they have done to me.
  [C/f/2,∗,i]

- Wept from seeing the movie "Maa-soom" (Innocent) even though I had seen it twice before. Felt about the little boy in the movie, that he was alone and had nowhere to go.
  [C/f/1,2/i]

- Threw away something I had been very fond of, on impulse, because it was slightly spoilt.
  [H/f/1,2/i]

- Did not want to eat or drink at a restaurant that I frequently visit, because I found it very dirty: because very particular about ironing clothes.
  [H/f/1,2/i]

- Usual lack of confidence was ameliorated.
  [C/f/2,∗/i]

- More confident than usual, while talking.
  [H/f/1,∗/i]

Intellect

- Was nervous and unable to concentrate on studies although I wanted to.
  [A/f/1,3/i]

- Concentration decreased.
  [D/f/1,3/i]

DREAMS

Future

■ I was sitting at the seashore, very tense about the future, my friends had an intercollegiate competition. Suddenly, I saw a saint near me, whom after a while I could recognize as Swami Vivekananda[1]. I was very happy to see him and felt sure that I would get good guidance for the future from him. He told me to live peacefully in the world. He asked me not to worry, saying that everything would be alright, God is great and would definitely help me in my future.

[A/m/1,7/i]

■ My Guru[2] was reading my palm and telling me that I would have a good future overall, but that there would still be some problems which I would have to face.

[B/m/2,2/i]

Fear

■ I was to be operated for appendicitis. I felt frightened and anxious before the operation and did not want to go through it. I kept praying to God to do something so that my operation continuously gets cancelled. And, at last, it was cancelled.

[D/f/1,1/i]

■ I was enjoying myself, playing with my family on the beach. Suddenly on one side of the beach the colour of the water changed from green to blue. Everyone went over to see it but they wouldn't allow me, saying that I would drown. I felt they wanted to leave me alone, but was also fearful of drowning. I wanted to enjoy myself with them.

[C/f/1,2/i]

■ I was driving my friend's car. I didn't know how to drive it, but she said I would

---

[1]   Indian philosopher.
[2]   Spiritual teacher; venerable person.

learn. I found it strange. Suddenly it became very small in size. But I continued to drive it. After sometime it began to rain and I parked the car in the premises of a building which were flooded with water. I was waiting for the rain to stop when someone screamed suddenly that there were snakes in the water. I looked behind me and saw two snakes – one gold and one black. I was very afraid that they would bite me and wanted to escape. I decided to leave immediately. Was terrified.

[F/f/1,1/i]

■ I have worn a dress with a black line on the right side. I don't pay any attention to it. Later, while undressing, I realize that the line was a dead, black snake. I start to scream and shout, and throw the dress away.

[F/f/2,∗/i]

■ I fall asleep while on the train, and miss my station. I get off at another station and want to catch another train back to my station. I see the ticket collector in front of me and am afraid because I do not have a ticket.

[I/m/1,5/i]

■ I suddenly found skin eruptions with severe itching and red discolouration all over my body. I was very much afraid. I feel, I look ugly.

[D/f/1,1/i]

■ I have an ugly ulcer on my right leg. I am very scared that I would look ugly with the ulcer. I cannot bear to look at it. I go to the doctor and ask him to amputate my leg. I feel I would rather die than have it.

[F/f/2,1/i]

Strange

■ I see strange people with heads divided into two parts; the top belonging to one person, and the bottom belonging to another person. I feel I am the odd man out, and I should get out of here.

[G/m/1,3/i]

- I was running about, here and there, without any purpose. I was running from a strange place that I had never seen before. I had the constant feeling that there was someone behind me, pursuing me. I came to a seashore. It was night time and there were strange people playing with a bat and ball. I felt strange and lonely. I was all alone and didn't know what to do.

[A/m/1,3/i]

- My close friend was in labour, and was having severe pains. But nothing came out after the contractions. Her husband was standing and smoking. He was not bothered, and wasn't upset, whatever had happened was okay with him. I found it odd; it was all very strange. I couldn't believe it. I felt sad for her. She expected something and something else had turned out.

Also, her husband looked very odd; he had a moustache. Looking at him I felt that time had passed, and I was more mature.

I felt guilty about dreaming something disastrous about such a close friend. She has always been helpful to me with my studies, and advises me regarding my behaviour.

[G/m/2,*/i]

- Two of my friends who were playing carrom asked me to join them. At first, I refused thinking I cannot play the game. Later I joined in and won with ease. I was happy to win. I felt even if I couldn't do anything the first time I could do it afterwards. It was a strange feeling.

[A/m/1,1/i]

Exams

- Dreams of exams.

[F/f/*,*/i]

- I was going for an exam when I suddenly wasn't sure whether I had my hall ticket.

I began to search in my purse but found the ticket from the last year. Then fifteen minutes before my exam, I rang up my college to ask whether they had my hall ticket.

I had to get to college but was unable to get a taxi. Then I asked a man with a hand cart for a lift and he obliged.

[E/f/1,3/i]

- I did not know any answers for an Organon exam that I was writing. I was upset, almost in tears, because I had decided to be amongst the rank-holders. A professor sat beside me and told me that I had scored one mark less than the minimum pass percentage. He shouted at me. I was extremely nervous and upset, and thought to myself why I was not able to reach my goal and get let down everytime even though I study so hard?

[F/f/1,2/i]

- I had gone to an Indian hill station with my mother and sister. I forgot to carry my books to study for an exam that was supposed to be held two days later. I was tense. We were staying in a very good hotel and there was a water fountain in our room. I was happy to see it. To my surprise I found Tulsi (*Ocimum sanctum*) leaves in the fountain.

[F/f/1,7/i]

Miscellaneous

- I was being taught by a very strict professor of whom we were very scared. But at the end of the lecture he taught us how to make an Indian snack and gave us some to taste. I liked it immensely and prepared the same on returning home. It turned out very well and everyone liked it very much.

[F/f/2,*/i]

- Cooking very spicy food and teaching others to cook.

[F/f/1,2/I]

- My mother is wearing some earrings. I feel they are new but she says that she has had them a long time. I feel she should've showed them to me earlier, and feel deceived.

[H/f/1,2/i]

▪ My father had died. I couldn't believe it. I was weeping continuously.

[F/f/2,2/i]

▪ I am travelling in a bus with a girl I like very much. I am surprised that a girl who normally doesn't talk to me is so friendly.

[I/m/1,4/i]

▪ I am playing cricket with my friends when two of them start to quarrel. I try to stop the fight as I do not like this, but am unable to stop it. I feel very sorry and nervous; they are my real friends yet I am unable to stop them.

[I/m/1,3/i]

▪ I suddenly noticed pustular eruptions coming up on my head while combing my hair. I was shocked. I cannot bear to see myself look so ugly.

[F/f/2,∗/i]

▪ I had to go for a cousin's wedding. The tailor hadn't got my dress ready. I tried many other dresses, but liked none. I was tense and upset and decided not to attend the wedding.

[F/f/4,4/i]

▪ I had gone for a pizza at a very big, crowded place. We were made to wait very long. There were two or three pregnant women who delivered there. I noticed that the gynaecologist sitting next to me had worn a necklace with two snake heads. I wanted to ask her why she had worn such a necklace.

[F/f/1,5/i]

▪ A professor had given us an exam to do. We were in a very big hall. Suddenly she gave us a break in which she had arranged a lunch party for us. I could see among the many food items, pizza coming out of the oven. Although I was very tempted to eat, I did not because I was tense about the exam we had to finish.

[F/f/1,6/i]

▪ My cousin got kidnapped. I managed to rescue her. My relatives were giving the credit to someone else who wasn't even present at the time. I was shocked and told everyone that I had done the job, but they wouldn't listen. I felt very bad that when I deserved the credit it was being given to someone else.

[F/f/1,3/i]

▪ Lascivious dream.

[F/f/1,4/i]

▪ I ask my professor if he will take a lecture, since it is a sacred day. He says he will.

[G/m/1,1,i]

▪ I see a girl in college. I do not want to talk to her. Feel that she should come and talk to me.

[G/m,1/1/i]

▪ A very drunk man is telling me that my friend has invited him home.

[G/m/1,4/i]

▪ I went to a wine shop with my friends and asked for scotch whisky. But it was very expensive, so I settled for a cheaper whisky. I found it surprising (since I don't drink). Happy, enjoyable.

[B/m/1,2/i]

▪ Fainting and falling again and again. My friends are around me.

[H/f/2,1/i]

▪ Dream about past birth.

[F/f/2,∗/i]

COINCIDENCE IN DR. RAJAN SANKARAN'S CLINIC ON 27.12.94

Three students of final year, from distant city, came and asked the following questions:

- In pregnant women is there one vital force or two vital forces?
- Should we give an anti-miasmatic remedy for the foetus?
- Can we use Acupuncture?
- Vaccination: is it there in Homoeopathy?

They asked me these questions with a lot of respect and wanted my opinion on these issues. I wanted to help, but did not want to spoon-feed my ideas in their minds. I wanted them to think for themselves and not to blindly stick to my way or ideas. I wanted to guide them on the way of thinking, for example: scientific thinking, practical thinking. I was rough with them, pushing their own questions back to themselves, making them think scientifically and logically at the same time, telling them my experiences. In the end, I myself offered them to conduct a course for them to orient themselves in a proper way. I was eager not to make them dependent on me completely, yet at the same time anxious that they should not be misguided. I had to be strict, at the same time not to be too strict but be kind and encouraging.

PHYSICAL SYMPTOMS

Generalities

- Craving for ice-cold water and cold drinks, every two hours.
  [A/m/1,2/i]
- Craving for sour, for example: buttermilk.
  [A/m/1,4/i]
- Thirst for cold water in small quantities, frequently.
  [B/m/1,5/i]
- Not tired, despite a lot of work.
  [C/f/1,4/i]
- Motion sickness very marked.
  [D/f/1,2/i]
- Craving for spicy food, ordinary food tasted very bland.
  [F/f/1,1/i]

- Craving for chillis.
  [F/f/2,*/i]
- Craving for pizza.
  [F/f/2,*/i]
- Weakness, and loss of appetite.
  [F/f/2,*/i]
- Chilly, could not bear slightest draft.
  [F/f/*,*/i]
- Decreased thirst.
  [H/f/1,1/i]
- Intense craving for cheese.
  [H/f/1,2/i]
- Craving for apples.
  [H/f/1,2/i]
- Feeling as if I am getting fatter, and

my clothes are too tight for me.
[H/f/1,3/i]
- Energetic, as if I have taken a tonic.
[H/f/1,3/i]
- Craving for buttermilk.
[H/f/*,*/i]

- Desire for covers.
[I/m/1,6/i]
- Desire for bitter things.
[J/m/1,2/i]

Physical particulars

Head

- Severe throbbing pain – temporal.
[A/m/before dose]
- Violent headache, not better from pressure. But better twenty minutes after hot drinks.
[B/m/1,2/i]
- Head pain in vertex.
[D/f/1,3/i]
- Throbbing pain in the frontal region and right temple with audible heart beats. Worse in the morning, on rising. Worse from light and motion. Better from closing the eyes, and at 12.30 p.m.
[F/f/2,*/i]
- Hairfall, tremendous, with fear.
[F/f/2,*/i]
- Severe throbbing, bursting pain.
[G/m/2,*/i]
- Throbbing headache – both temples and frontal region. Began in the morning. Gradually the intensity would increase until it was severe at night. Accompanied by nausea. Aggravated from light, motion, hairbath, cold air, perfume, noise. Ameliorated from extending the neck, closing eyes, pressure, evening, night.
[F/f/3,*/i]
- Dull, electric current-like headache lasting two-three minutes, on taking the dose. Throbbing in frontal region.
[H/f/1,1/i]
- Usual hairfall has stopped.
[H/f/2,3/i]

- Throbbing pain in frontal region.
[I/m/2,*/i]
- Cold perspiration following exertion.
[I/m/1,1/i]
- Throbbing pain in frontal region.
[G/m/1,1/i]

Eyes

- Heaviness in the eyes, with sleepiness.
[B/m/1,5/i]
- Itching in the right eye in the morning.
[C/f/1,1/i]
- Intense itching in the left eye at night, with burning. Better by applying cold water.
[C/f/1,1/i]
- Lachrymation and itching in both the eyes in the morning.
[C/f/1,3/i]
- Pulsating sensation in the eye.
[E/f/2,*/ii]
- Burning from overuse. Worse closing the eyes. Better from washing.
[I/m/1,2/i]

Nose

- Sneezing; five-six sneezes at a time. Watery, bland discharge.
[A/m/1,2/i]
- Right-sided nose block.
[A/m/1,2/i]
- Nasal block, on waking in the morning.
[B/m/1,1/i]

- Block in the right nostril, on waking in the morning.

  [B/m/1,2/i]

- Sneezing aggravated in the mornings. Coryza: yellow-white, watery.

  [I/m/1,5/i]

- Right-sided nasal block on waking in the morning, later shifting to the left side.

  [B/m/1,3/i]

- Watery coryza.

  [B/m/1,6/i]

- Coryza aggravated between 7.00 p.m. and 8.00 p.m.

  [B/m/2,1/i]

- Watery coryza.

  [D/f/1,3/i]

- Left nostril stopped up at night, during sleep. Aggravated uncovering even a single part of the body.

  [I/m/1,1/i]

Face

- Cold perspiration following exertion.

  [I/m/1,1/i]

Mouth

- Tip of the tongue was sensitive to touch.

  [C/f/1,4/i]

Throat

- Sensation of mucus plug in the throat which I wanted to expectorate, but was unable to.

  [B/m/1,2/i]

- Dryness in the throat, with thirst for small quantities of water, frequently.

  [B/m/1,5/i]

- Pain while swallowing.

  [C/f/2,*/i]

- Wanted to keep something cold in the throat.

  [B/m/2,6/i]

- Sensation as if there is something stuck in the throat, which must be removed.

  [I/m/1,6/i]

- Irritation in the throat, ameliorated from warmth.

  [I/m/1,5/i]

- Pain while swallowing. Swallowing liquids is less painful than swallowing solids. Better from warm drinks. Worse from cold air, cold drinks. Worse morning and evening.

  [F/f/2,*/i]

- Pain, worse empty swallowing.

  [J/m/1,2/i]

External throat

- Cold perspiration following exertion.

  [I/m/1,1/i]

Stomach

- Pain and heaviness in the stomach. Feeling of fullness in the stomach after having eaten a small quantity.

  [C/f/2,3/i]

- Thirst for large quantities, at long intervals.

  [I/m/1,2/i]

- Appetite very much increased; can eat again after a full meal.

  [A/m/1,4/i]

- Increased appetite with decreased thirst.

  [D/f/1,2/i]

- Increased appetite in spite of full stomach, but no hunger.

  [H/f/1,1/i]

- Appetite increased; desire to eat all the time.

  [H/f/1,3/i]

- Decreased thirst.

  [H/f/1,1/i]

Abdomen

- Abdominal pain at 11.30 p.m., lasting for nearly one hour. Aggravated from sitting and walking. Ameliorated from sleeping.

[B/m/1,2/i]

- Severe pain in the abdomen, worse at night between 4.00 a.m. and 5.00 a.m. Better from hot drinks.

[C/f/1,4/i]

- Pulsation in epigastrium, on taking the dose.

[H/f/1,1/i]

- Feeling as if there was a hard pad in the epigastrium, after eating.

[H/f/1,2/i]

- Severe cramping in abdomen during menses.

[D/f/2,*/i]

- Heaviness as from a stone in epigastrium, after eating.

[H/f/1,3/i]

- Cutting pain in the epigastrium. Worse from pressure.

Rectum

- Pain during and after stool.

[I/m/1,1/i]

- Urge to stool after eating.

[I/m/1,1/i]

Stool

- Dry stool, difficulty in passing stool.

[G/m/*,*/i]

- Flatus before stool.

[B/m/2,5/i]

- Dry cough in the daytime.

[I/m/1,6/i]

Bladder

- Frequency of urination at night.

[D/f/1,1/i]

Cough

- Mild cough in the morning and at night.

[D/ f1,1/i]

- Cough, worse from talking.

[E/f/1,3/i]

- Violent, continuous cough. Lasts twenty minutes at a time.

[I/m/2,*/i]

Expectoration

- White, watery sputum.

[B/m/1,5/i]

- Difficult, white, sweetish.

[E/ /1,3/i]

- Expectoration only at night.

[I/m/1,6/i]

- Dry, thick, in the evening.

[J/m/1,2/i]

Chest

- Burning in the sternal region.

[C/f/2,3/i]

- Palpitation from least exertion.

[I/m/1,2/i]

- Palpitations aggravated lying on left side.

[J/m/1,2/i]

Extremities

- Numbness of the left limb, mainly in the morning, ameliorated from motion.

[A/m/1,2/i]

- Severe pain in the thigh during menses. Worse at night. Recurred after eight days.

[D/f/1,4/i]

- Weak and insecure feeling in the joints especially of the lower limbs. Painful to walk further.

[H/f/1,2/i]

- Continuous pain in the left foot. Want to stand on the front part of the foot. Ameliorated from lying down.

[I/m/1,5/i]

- Repeated sprains in the legs, especially left knee joint.

[H/f/1,3/i]

- Itching in the hips (old symptom reappeared). Better from cold.

[I/m/1,1/i]

- Pain lower limbs, on walking. Desire for complete rest.

[I/m/1,3/i]

- Throbbing pain, right hip joint. Aggravated from motion, pressure. Ameliorated from rest.

[I/m/1,4/i]

- Twitching of muscles in left upper and lower extremities.

[F/f/1,*/i]

Sleep

- Very sleepy one hour before the usual bedtime, almost immediately after dinner.

[A/m/1,6/i]

- Sleepiness.

[B/m/1,5/i]

- Tired and sleepy in the afternoon, but was unable to sleep. Was turning from side to side before finally getting to sleep. Woke up from a very slight noise.

[C/f/1,1/i]

- Drowsy throughout the day.

[F/f/1,1/i]

- Unusually fresh and energetic on waking.

[H/f/1,1/i]

RUBRICS

Mind

Single symptoms
— Company, desire for, friend, of a faithful.

— Delusion, a hand behind him.

— Dreams, alone, of being.

— Dreams, anxious, quarrels, friends, between.

— Dreams, body, body parts, head, pustular eruptions on.

— Dreams, body, body parts, ulcer, right leg, on.

— Dreams, car, learning to drive.

— Dreams, car, shrinking.

— Dreams, credit, she deserved, being given to someone else.

— Dreams, deceived.

— Dreams, food, pizza.

— Dreams, future, being told.

— Dreams, game, playing, a new.

— Dreams, game, refusing to join in from want of confidence, which he later won with ease.

— Dreams, guided, being.

— Dreams, guidance seeking.

— Dreams, mature, of being.

— Dream, people, strange, with heads divided into two.

— Dreams, learning to cook.

— Dreams, praying anxiously before her surgery.

— Dreams, saints.

— Dreams, strange place, being in.

— Dreams, ugly, of being.

— Faith and friendship, need to maintain.

— Guidance, need for.

Common symptoms
— Abusive, insulting.

— Ailments, from anger, suppressed.

— Amusement, desire for.

— Anger, noise, from.

— Anxiety, future, about.

— Company, aversion to, aggravates.

— Company, aversion to, solitude, fond of.

— **Company, desire for**.

— Concentration, difficult.

— Contradiction, aggravates.

— Delusion, neglected.

— Delusion, people, sees someone behind him.

— Dreams, animals, snakes, of.

— Dreams, anxious.

— Dreams, death, father.

— Dreams, death, relatives.

— Dreams, disease.

— Dreams, disease, loathsome

— Dreams, eruptions.

— Dreams, fainting.

— Dreams, food.

— *Dreams, frightful.*

— Dreams, lewd, lascivious, voluptuous.

— Dreams, pursued, being.

— Dreams, running.

— *Dreams, strange.*

— Dreams, water, danger from.

— Fear, dark, of.

— Fear, happen, something will.

— Fear, new persons, of.
— Fear, robbers, of.
— Fear, strangers, of.
— Fear, undertaking, new enterprise, a.
— Forsaken feeling.
— Irritability, noise, from.
— Irritability, trifles, at.
— Malicious.
— Music, ameliorates.

— Restlessness.
— Restlessness, afternoon, 4 p.m.
— Rudeness.
— Sadness, melancholy, future, about the.
— Selfishness, egoism.
— Sensitive, oversensitive, noise, to.
— **Starting, startled**.
— Starting, startled, easily.

PHYSICAL SYMPTOMS

Generalities

–   Air, draft, of, aggravates.
–   Cold, aggravates.
–   Covers, ameliorates, and desire for.
–   Food, apples, desires.
–   Food, buttermilk, desires.
–   Food, cheese, desires.
–   Food, cold drink, cold water desires.
–   Food, pizza, desires (single).
–   Food, pungent, desires.
–   Food, sour, desires.
–   Food, spices, desires.
–   Motion aggravates.
–   Strength, sensation of.
–   Twitching.
–   Twitching, one-sided.
–   Twitching, one-sided, left (single).
–   Weakness.

Head

–   Hair, falling.
–   **Pain**.
–   Pain, violent pains.
–   Pain, drinks, warm, ameliorates.
–   Pain, vertex.

–   Perspiration, cold.
–   **Pulsating**.
–   Pulsating, temples.
–   *Pulsating, forehead*.
–   Pulsating, temple, right.
–   Pulsating, morning, rising, on.
–   Pulsating, accompanied by palpitations (single).
–   Pulsating, light aggravates.
–   Pulsating, motion aggravates.
–   Pulsating, closing eyes ameliorates (single).
–   Pulsating, noon ameliorates (single).
–   Pulsating, morning.
–   Pulsating, nausea, with (single).
–   Pulsating, bathing, after.
–   Pulsating, cold air.
–   Pulsating, odours, from.
–   Pulsating, extending the neck ameliorates (single).
–   Pulsating, pressure ameliorates.
–   Pulsating, noise, from.
–   Pulsating, evening ameliorates (single).

Eye
- Heaviness.
- Itching.
- Itching, right (single).
- Itching, left.
- Itching, morning.
- Itching, night.
- Itching, cold water ameliorates (single).
- Lachrymation, morning.
- Pain, burning.
- Pain, burning, cold bathing ameliorates.
- Pain, burning, closing lids.
- Pain, pulsating.

Nose
- Coryza, evening, 7.00 p.m.- 8.00 p.m. (single).
- Discharge, bland.
- Discharge, watery.
- Obstruction, one side.
- Obstruction, right.
- Obstruction, right, then left.
- Obstruction, left.
- Obstruction, morning, waking, on.
- Obstruction, night.
- Obstruction, left side, uncovering any part of the body aggravates (single).
- Sneezing, morning.
- Sneezing, paroxysmal.

Face
- Perspiration, cold.

Mouth
- Sensitive, tongue.
- Sensitive, tongue tip.

Throat
- Dryness.
- Foreign body, sensation of a.

- Irritation, warmth ameliorates (single).
- Pain, morning.
- Pain, evening.
- Pain, air cold aggravages.
- Pain, drinks, cold aggravates.
- Pain, drinks, warm ameliorates.
- Pain, swallowing.
- Pain, swallowing food.

External throat
- Perspiration – cold (single).

Stomach
- *Appetite, increased.*
- Fullness, eating, ever, so little, after.
- Heaviness.
- Pain.
- Thirst, large quantities, for, and often.
- Heaviness.
- Pain.

Abdomen
- Fullness, sensation of, eating, after.
- Heaviness, as from a load.
- Pain.
- Pain, noon.
- Pain, night.
- Pain, bending double ameliorates.
- Pain, pressure aggravates.
- Pain, sitting, while.
- Pain, sleep aggravates.
- Pain, walking, while.

Rectum
- Flatus, stool, before.
- Pain.
- Pain, stool, during.
- Pain, stool, after.
- Urging.
- Urging, eating, after.

Stool
- Dry.
- Hard.

Bladder
- Urination, frequent, night.

Cough
- Morning.
- Night.
- Dry.
- Dry, daytime.
- Talking.

Expectoration
- Night.
- Dry,
- Dry, day time.
- Talking.

Chest
- Pain, burning, sternum.
- Palpitation.

- Palpitation, exertion, least, from the.

Extremities
- Injuries, ankle.
- Itching, nates.
- Itching, nates, cold aggravates (single).
- Numbness, morning.
- *Pain, lower limbs*.
- Pain, lower limbs, night.
- Pain, hip, motion, aggravates.
- Pain, hip, pressure aggravates (single).
- Pain, sprained as if, ankle.
- Pulsation, hip.
- Weakness, joints.
- Weakness, lower limbs.

Sleep
- Sleepiness.
- Sleepiness, afternoon.
- Sleeplessness, sleepiness with, daytime.

THEMES

1. **Desire for company, especially friends**
   Feeling he needs the faith of his friends, and he must not break this faith.
   Feeling unwanted by friends, cheated by friends and desire for one faithful friend.
   Feeling he can understand his friends' problems, and is always in contact with a friend in trouble.

2. **Desire for guidance from professors, learned persons, gurus**
   Feels he has some support behind him.
   Praying to God to help her in crisis.

3. **Fears**
   Future, profession.
   Being alone.
   Someone behind her, following her.
   Of being harmed.
   Competition, anticipatory.
   Drowning.
   Operation.
   Snakes.
   Happen, something will.

4. Refusing to join in a new game from want of confidence.

5. Death of father.

6. Strange place.
   Strange people.
   Strange feeling.
   Strange happenings.

7. **Irritability**
   Suppressed.
   Noise from, talk of others.
   Contradiction.
   Trifles.
   Family, with.
   Friends being selfish.

8. Wanting to enjoy themselves, watch movies, visit different places, spend money.
   Unable to concentrate on studies, work.

9. Restlessness.

10. Desire to be alone.

11. Music, dancing.

12. Selfish.

13. Ugly – skin eruptions.

14. Driving car.
    Dance competition.
    New game.
    New profession.
    Examinations.
    Learning to cook.